"Well, Mary Brady has done it yet again. This is a beautiful book, full of tumult, turbulence, bravery and grace. The clinical work is outstanding, and the image of surfing is the most apt we clinicians have ever been provided with for adolescent treatment. I used to think of tightropes, but surfing takes you forward to some-where – maybe even somewhere thrilling."

**Anne Alvarez**, *PhD, MACP, Consultant Child and Adolescent Psychotherapist*

"In publishing this book, Mary Brady invites us to embark on a journey, and she does so with a skill that can only be acquired through years of clinical practice, deep reflection, and experience in writing and publishing in psychoanalysis. This excellent book invites us to surf its pages, glide through them, and share the exciting experience of analyzing adolescents – the true protagonists of all the significant historical changes ahead."

**Virginia Ungar**, *MD, Past President of the International Psychoanalytic Association (2017 – 2021)*

"Based on her clinical expertise with children and adolescents, Mary T. Brady's book captures the essence and the complexity of psychoanalytic technique with young patients who are in pain and in severely damaged environments. The book includes beautiful chapters, some in collaboration with other eminent psychoanalysts. The diversity of clinical work presented here and the rigor of theory, for instance in the usage of Wilfred Bion and Donald Winnicott makes this book stand out. I have no doubt that it will be of great interest to those working in the field of mental health."

**Christine Anzieu-Premmereur**, *MD, PhD, Chair of the IPA Committee on Child and Adolescent Psychoanalysis*

# Psychoanalysis with Adolescents and Children

In *Psychoanalysis with Adolescents and Children: Learning to Surf*, Mary T. Brady expertly guides the reader through the challenging and vital process of working with young analysands.

Brady likens the experience to 'learning to surf.' While finding Bion's metaphor that the analyst must be able to 'think under fire' useful, she suggests 'learning to surf' is more apt in psychoanalysis with adolescents and children. Drawing on this metaphor throughout the volume, she describes how the adolescent can be potentially upended, injured or even killed by emotional waves too tumultuous to manage. Surfing also evokes the often uneasy but sometimes thrilling balances of adolescence. Using clinical vignettes from her extensive experience in the field, Brady explores how to work with young people experiencing issues such as eating disorders, gender challenges, parental substance abuse and the impact of the COVID-19 pandemic. Drawing on Bionian Field Theory, as well as the work of Donald Winnicott, she explores how analysts can surf with the adolescent or child in navigating the ebb and flow of psychic life and development.

This book is essential reading for psychoanalysts and psychotherapists, including psychiatrists, psychologists, therapists and counselors, who treat children and adolescents.

**Mary T. Brady** is an adult and child psychoanalyst in San Francisco, USA. On the Faculties of the San Francisco Center for Psychoanalysis and the Psychoanalytic Institute of Northern California, she is a recipient of the American Psychoanalytic Association's Roughton Award for her writing. She is the editor of *Braving the Erotic Field in the Treatment of Children and Adolescents* (2022) and the author of *Analytic Engagements with Adolescents* (2018) and *The Body in Adolescence* (2015). She is Co-Chair for the Committee on Child and Adolescent Psychoanalysis (COCAP) of the IPA and has co-led a *Psychoanalysis and Film* group for a decade.

# Routledge Child and Adolescent Psychoanalysis

Editor: Christine Anzieu-Premmereur
Co-Editors: Mary T. Brady
Christine Franckx
Fernando Gomez

The Routledge Child and Adolescent Psychoanalysis Book Series is devoted to manuscripts that illuminate the creative and challenging work of child and adolescent psychoanalysis and psychoanalytic psychotherapy. While we believe that the study of child psychoanalysis is relevant to all psychoanalysts – as the study of the unconscious is essential to all psychoanalysts – the particularities of child and adolescent work require that the setting adapt itself to the child and adolescent, not the other way around. We also see children and adolescents as quite sensitive to cultural and societal changes and catastrophes. Children and adolescents are like the canaries in the coal mine – particularly vulnerable to the presence of gases. For that reason, our Book Series is dedicated to excellent and creative clinical technique and theoretical work, writing that is sensitive to the setting, and writing that is perceptive of societal and cultural changes that affect children and adolescents.

The series editors are especially interested in selecting books which enhance the understanding and further expansion of infant, child, and adolescent psychoanalytic thought. Part of the mission of this international series is to nurture communication amongst psychoanalysts working in different models, in different languages, and in different regions of the world.

## Series Editor Biographies

**Christine Anzieu-Premmereur** is a psychiatrist and psychoanalyst in New York City who works in private practice with adults, children, parents and their babies. A member of the Société Psychanalytique de Paris, she is on the faculty of the Columbia Psychoanalytic Center for Training and Research and is Assistant Clinical Professor in Psychiatry at Columbia University. She is the chair of the IPA Committee for Child and Adolescent Psychoanalysis (COCAP). With Vaia Tsolas, she is the co-founder of Pulsion Institute. She recently published *The Process of Representation in Early Childhood* and *Attacks on Linking in Parents of Young Disturbed Children*. She co-edited with Vaia Tsolas *A Psychoanalytic Exploration of the Body in Today's World: On the Body* (2017) and *A Psychoanalytic Exploration of the Contemporary Search for Pleasure: The Turning of the Screw* (2023).

**Dr. Mary T. Brady** is an adult and child psychoanalyst in private practice in San Francisco, USA. She is on the Faculties of the San Francisco Center for Psychoanalysis and the Psychoanalytic Institute of Northern California. She is Editor of *Braving the Erotic Field in the Treatment of Children and Adolescents* (2022). Her books, *Analytic Engagements with Adolescents* and *The Body in Adolescence* were published by Routledge in 2018 and 2016 respectively. She is North American Co-Chair for the Committee on Child and Adolescent Psychoanalysis (COCAP) of the IPA. She co-leads a Psychoanalysis and Film group.

**Dr. Christine Franckx** is an adult and child psychoanalyst and psychiatrist. She works in Antwerp in private practice for adult analysis and she has created an analytic psychotherapeutic center for early development (0–6 years). She is a Training Analyst of the Belgian Psychoanalytic Society, of which she has been the President (2016–2020). She is Editor of two books *Eros op de scene* (2021) and *Het kinderlijk trauma* (2023). She is trainer in Infant observation (Esther Bick). She is European Co-Chair for the IPA Committee on Child and Adolescent Psychoanalysis (COCAP).

**Dr. Fernando M. Gómez** is a child and adolescent psychoanalyst, psychiatrist and pediatrician. He works in Buenos Aires in private practice for children, adolescents and adults analysis. He was trained at the Asociación Psicoanalítica Argentina (APA), of which he has been Director of the Publications Committee (2016–2020) and of the Department of Children and Adolescents "Arminda Aberastury" (2020–2023). He is Latin American Co-Chair for the IPA Committee for Child and Adolescent Psychoanalysis (COCAP). He is a member of the Advisory Council of the General Directorate of Mental Health of the Government of the City of Buenos Aires. He edited a 4 volumes collection: *Pilares del Psicoanálisis Contemporáneo* (2017, 2018, 2019, 2020), *Psicoanálisis Contemporáneo Latinoamericano* (2017, coedited with FEPAL), and he is currently editing *Clinica e Investigación en el Psicoanalisis de bebés, niños y adolescentes. Nuevos horizontes, nuevos desafíos.*

## Forthcoming Titles

### Psychoanalysis with Adolescents and Children
Learning to Surf
*Mary T. Brady*

# Psychoanalysis with Adolescents and Children

## Learning to Surf

Mary T. Brady

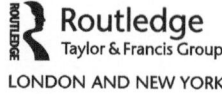

Routledge
Taylor & Francis Group

LONDON AND NEW YORK

Designed cover image: Getty © Westend61

First published 2025
by Routledge
4 Park Square, Milton Park, Abingdon, Oxon OX14 4RN

and by Routledge
605 Third Avenue, New York, NY 10158

*Routledge is an imprint of the Taylor & Francis Group, an informa business*

© 2025 Mary T. Brady

*British Library Cataloguing-in-Publication Data*
A catalogue record for this book is available from the British
Library

ISBN: 978-1-032-81243-4 (hbk)
ISBN: 978-1-032-76519-8 (pbk)
ISBN: 978-1-003-49881-0 (ebk)

DOI: 10.4324/9781003498810

Typeset in Times New Roman
by Apex CoVantage, LLC

For Jacquie, Dawn and Sharon

# Contents

# Series Foreword

The Committee on Child and Adolescent Psychoanalysis (COCAP) is delighted to present this first book in our new Series – *Psychoanalysis with Adolescents and Children: Learning to Surf* by Mary T. Brady. Based on her clinical expertise with children and adolescents, Mary T. Brady's book captures the essence and the complexity of psychoanalytic technique with young patients who are in pain and in severely damaged environments. The book includes beautiful chapters, some in collaboration with other eminent psychoanalysts. The diversity of clinical work presented here and the rigor of theory, for instance in the usage of Wilfred Bion and Donald Winnicott makes this book stand out. I have no doubt that it will be of great interest to those working in psychoanalysis and in mental health in general.

The COCAP Book Series is devoted to manuscripts that illuminate the creative and challenging work of child and adolescent psychoanalysis and psychoanalytic psychotherapy. While we believe that the study of child psychoanalysis is relevant to all psychoanalysts – as the study of the unconscious is essential to all psychoanalysts – the particularities of child and adolescent work require that the setting adapt itself to the child and adolescent, not the other way around. We see children and adolescents as quite sensitive to cultural and societal changes and catastrophes. Children and adolescents are like the canaries in the coal mine – particularly vulnerable to the presence of gases. For that reason, our Book Series is dedicated to excellent and creative clinical technique and theoretical work, writing that is sensitive to the setting, and writing that is perceptive of societal and cultural changes that affect children and adolescents.

The series editors are especially interested in selecting books which enhance the understanding and further expansion of infant, child, and adolescent psychoanalytic thought. A mission of this international series is to nurture communication amongst psychoanalysts working in different models, in different languages, and in different regions of the world.

Series Editor: Christine Anzieu-Premmereur

Chair, Committee on Child and Adolescent Psychoanalysis

# Foreword

In the broad and complex field of psychoanalysis, practice with adolescents stands out for its uniqueness, its capacity to generate intense emotionality in the analytic couple, and the challenge it presents.

In publishing this book, Mary T. Brady invites us to embark on a journey, and she does so with a skill that can only be acquired through years of clinical practice, deep reflection, and experience in writing and publishing in psychoanalysis.

In this sense, from her position as Chair for North America of the Committee on Child and Adolescent Psychoanalysis (COCAP) of the International Psychoanalytic Association, she inaugurates its new Routledge book series with this – its first book.

Already from the title of this book, she offers an exceptional metaphor in the act of surfing. Surfing involves the body in search of balance, displacement on a moving water floor that requires precise timing, and the feeling of ecstasy if one manages to stay on the highest point of the wave. All this, together with the fear of an imminent leap into the void and a lack of precision about the point of arrival.

Adolescence is a time of surfing in a whirlwind of emotions in which both the analyst and the patient are immersed, facing waves that can be tumultuous, threatening imbalance, or drowning. Also, following Bion and learning from experience, adolescents encounter the thrill of adventure and the feeling of being fully alive together. In my experience, nothing could compare to the vitality, the desire to know, and the commitment to the task that prevails in working with adolescents in an analysis in which the transference-countertransference relationship is sustained and produces novelty.

Brady tells us that she relies on Bion for his theoretical clinical developments. In his article "Emotional Turbulence" (1976), this brilliant author refers to puberty and uses art to illustrate his ideas by referring to Leonardo da Vinci's drawings in which water swirls tumultuously as does hair in disorder. Bion uses these specific images to evoke in readers those periods of mental turmoil and turbulence *in themselves* and so attune them to what is happening with pubescent patients.

Brady's developments also incorporate the Barangers' field theory. This helps her address the transference-countertransference relationship and the deep involvement of patients and analysts in analytic work with young people.

In this sense, it is understandable that the book begins with a reflection on her personal history, trying to think about the origins of her vocation to treat adolescents. She does so in a way that is both sincere and moving for the reader.

Moreover, experience in the analytic treatment of children runs through every chapter of the book. Nothing touches the analyst's infantile structures more than the analysis of adolescents. They are more focused on the external world and have little willingness to 'look inwards.' Here, the practice with children that enhances the work with patients of any age comes to the rescue because it helps to make contact with the more primitive layers of mental life and the nonverbal levels of language.

Mary T. Brady especially highlights the importance of play in children's analysis by reminding us that play is both a physical and verbal expression of emotions and that in an analytic process, the experience of playing together is as vital as the interpretations that arise from it.

Throughout the chapters, Brady takes us on a journey as varied as it is enjoyable for all professionals working with adolescents. She presents us with a series of clinical situations that address a wide range of issues, from complex family relationships affected by alcoholism to gender dynamics in adolescence. The book also devotes significant space to the interaction between the individual and his or her environment, as it appears in references to the COVID-19 pandemic and the influence of totalitarian regimes on the minds of children.

Of particular note is the presentation of the oblivious object in the third chapter, which represents an essential contribution to post-Kleinian object relations theory. This chapter explores the complex dynamics between children and their parental figures, highlighting how children's conscious and unconscious perceptions of parental objects influence how they perceive and relate to the world around them. This chapter explores the distinction between a child's relationship with a 'stupid object' conceptualized by Anne Alvarez. In this case, the child has no concept of an intelligent object, i.e., one with an interested and interesting mind. On the other hand, children who relate to an "oblivious object" may consciously perceive their parents as intelligent and successful but unconsciously experience that they are not connected to the child's emotional needs. The transference-countertransference relationship may allow the beginning of a sense of an object that may be genuinely useful to the child. To exemplify these vicissitudes, the chapter includes material from the analyses of a late adolescent male and a 13-year-old girl.

Reading this volume is indispensable in trying to understand and help adolescents whose developmental task is to make the migration from the world of childhood to participation in a broader culture. The world we are living in these days post-pandemic, coupled with the climatic tragedy and wars, is not inviting for young people. We see the consequences of this situation in our clinical practice. However, adolescents go forward when they can, thirsty for knowledge, vital, creative, and passionate. When they are interested in their inner world, emotions, and dreams and meet an analyst who is receptive, sincere, and open to producing novelties, the experience can be wonderful.

This excellent book invites us to surf its pages, glide through them, and share the exciting experience of analyzing adolescents – the true protagonists of all the significant historical changes ahead.

Virginia Ungar
Past President of the IPA (2017–2021)

# Permissions

Chapter One was first published as:

Brady, M.T. (2022). Learning to surf: Analyzing adolescents. In J. Salberg (ed.) *Psychoanalytic Credos: Personal and Professional Journeys of Psychoanalysts. (pp. 155–159)*. London and New York: Routledge.

Chapter Two was first published as:

Brady, M.T. (2021). "Daddy's Head is Broken": The Treatment of Children of Severe Alcoholics. *Psychoanalytic Study of the Child*, 74, 234–248.

Chapter Three was first published as:

Brady, M.T. (2022). The oblivious object. In N. Parada Franche, C. Anzieu- Premmereur, M. Cardenal & M. Winberg Salomonsson (eds.) *The Infinite Infantile and the Psychoanalytic Task: Psychoanalyis with Children, Adolescents and Their Families*, Chapter 3, (pp. 36–48). Routledge.

Chapter Four was first published as:

Molinari, E. and Brady, M.T. (2022). Adolescent feminine subjectivities elaborated via transitory objects created in the analytic field. *Journal of Infant, Child, and Adolescent Psychotherapy*, 21(1), 60–71.

Chapter Six was first published as:

Brady, M., Tyminski, R. and Carey, K. (2012). To know or not to know: an application of Bion's K and –K to child treatment. *Journal of Child Psychotherapy*, 38(3), 302–317.

An earlier version of Chapter Seven was first published as:

Brady, M.T. (2021). Bazi Anoreksiya Vakalarinda Gorulen Bir Ergenlik Duslemic: Anneyi Yiyip Bitirme Korkusu, (An adolescent fantasy in some cases of anorexia: Fear of eating up the mother). In (ed. Tijen Demirors) *Siddet ve Yikicilik* (*Violence and Destruction)*, (pp. 137–144).

Part of Chapter Eight was first published as:

Brady, M.T. (2023) Règims totalitaris i una ment infantil: *Cría cuervos*. Revista Catalana de Psicoanàlisi, Vol. XL/2.

# Introduction

## Psychoanalysis with Adolescents and Children: Learning to Surf

I can think of no better image to capture the risks and joys of adolescence, or the risks and joys of treating adolescents, than surfing. As analysts, we are often immersed in languages of pathology or disturbance. Surfing evokes the dangers or even catastrophes of adolescence, but especially the exhilaration. It is too easy, even defensive, for analysts to speak of dangers. What of the thrills? What of young bodies finding their way? What of being noticed by that boy or that girl? What of something that just feels right? What of dancing until well into the morning? What of driving one's car a little too fast with the music on loud? As Winnicott (known for his interest in health) says, "[W]ith the proviso that adults do not abdicate, we may surely think of the strivings of adolescents to find themselves and determine their own destiny as the most exciting thing we can see in life around us" (1971, 146–147). As an analyst, I am also acutely aware of the dangers – of adolescents who wipe out on walls of water they thought they could ride.

Winnicott and Bion[1] are the theorists I rely on most in this book. In the chapters that follow, each will come forward often, along with other great theorists, including Melanie Klein and Henri Rey.

Regarding Bion, I often think of his aphorisms that the only thing of importance in a clinical hour is the unknown, as well as that 'the analyst must be able to think under fire.'

Yet, the metaphor of 'learning to surf' is more fundamental to the experience of adolescent and child analysis (than thinking under fire) when development itself leads to a lack of equilibrium and stability. A greater element of mobility is required in the analyst than in work with adults, with adolescents for whom action is the mode of being.

Regarding Winnicott, I often think of his emphasis on the spontaneous gesture in the child or adolescent (instead of conformity leading to false self) (Winnicott & Rodman, 1987), as well as his emphasis on the development of the capacity for play. Winnicott was particularly interested in *environments* that allow spontaneity in the child or adolescent to flourish. Ideally, adolescents are absorbed with discovering *themselves* and not us – they need us there but in the background. His concept of 'the doldrums' (2007/1968) conveys the need for development to take its own time – change can only be absorbed so fast. I also find Winnicott's concept of the

DOI: 10.4324/9781003498810-1

'antisocial tendency' in adolescence to be crucial, particularly his: "understanding that the antisocial act is an expression of hope" (1975/1958, 309).

Ogden (2024) describes a shift in psychoanalysis from an epistemological orientation (coming to understand) epitomized by Freud and Klein to an ontological orientation (coming into being) articulated by Bion and Winnicott. He suggests that in both late Bion and late Winnicott, the analyst's role is to help the patient creatively discover meaning for herself, in that way, becoming increasingly alive. For whom could this be more true than for adolescents? Adolescents need to put us in the background because what matters is that they are alive and that what they are doing is real and vivid. Even their hate and destructiveness – hard as it can be for us to bear – can lead to growth if it involves real contact with themselves and evokes a response in a parent or analyst that means something. They want adults out of the way, and yet they need us to provide a holding environment for their 'going on being,' to provide brakes when they go too fast as well as to rescue them when they crash.

How to live in one's own body – unlike any other body – is a central challenge for children and adolescents. How do I live with this skin color, this natal genitalia, this weight, this shape, this sense of bodily attractiveness, this sense of a body working well or malfunctioning? Adolescents and children are absorbing many other things as well – how do I live in this economic circumstance, with this level of privilege or deprivation, with these differences from my peers, etc.?

## Adolescents

I will speak first of adolescents because the metaphor of surfing is most apt with them.

While adolescence is a developmental phase, I would also suggest it is a state – the state of being on edge, neither falling back for too long into the old and familiar nor escaping the instability by foreclosing, for instance, into a too quickly adopted adult identity. Neither completely forgoing experimentation nor crashing into self-destruction. Anderson and Dartington suggest,

> [I]t seems to be those young people who have the inner strength and resources to bear to continue the experience of being naturally out of balance, as well as an environment that can support this, who "can achieve the best adjustment in adult life."
>
> (1998, 3)

The adolescent is faced with experiencing an otherness internally, 'I am no longer in the body I had as a child.' Adolescents are dislodged constantly from acquired positions, with only occasional resting places. In life, our resting places are body/mind situations in which we have some sense of stability and identity – 'this is me.' These resting states are disturbed throughout life. How does one apprehend emerging from a child's body to a pubertal body, from a healthy body to a sick or injured one, from life to an apprehension of death? Entry into puberty from the safer land of latency is such a dislodgement.

The body in adolescence emerges in relation to a mind that is not yet ready to process its impact. That which exceeds the capacity to process – the not yet representable (see Puget, 2016) – often leads to projective identification, which leaves the analyst feeling turned upside down and disoriented, or more problematically, to symptoms expressed through the adolescent's body (Brady, 2016).

Adolescents try things on and see how they fit – often in exaggerated form. The becoming of adolescence can yield intensities and instabilities that feel isolating and inexplicable. Augoyard uses the concept of 'hyperbole' in adolescence to designate a "violent over-exaggeration" that forces the object to struggle with "the painful and unbearable unknown emotional territory to be discovered (dark night pain)" (2023, 2). By "dark night" pain, she is referring to Bion's assertion that "becoming" is felt as inseparable from becoming God . . . the 'dark night' pain is "fear of megalomania" (Bion, 1965).

I will give a brief vignette to convey this rigidified, hyperbolic persona that masks a 'dark night pain.' 'Stephen,' an exceptionally intelligent 18-year-old analytic patient, had frank ideas of being God. This yielded intense loneliness as, in this state of mind, others were insignificant – an arrogant but agonizing dark night. Stephen required me to be an audience. He needed me as an audience, but the need could not be acknowledged to a degree that was close to annihilative. In such an annihilative moment, I confronted him, saying that "he lived in a world of one." This challenge got through, and Stephen has come back to my comment several times, showing that a second mind begins to come in and soften the hyperbolic self.

An adult patient could also be isolated in a highly narcissistic state. However, in adolescence, there can be something of an extreme to this. The adolescent is rightly flexing newfound muscles – for Stephen, his truly unusual intellectual acuity. However, his hyperbolic brilliance was matched only by his hyperbolic lack of emotional development – leading to a highly unstable mix. Following my confrontation with him, Stephen spoke compellingly of his terror of mental breakdown.

While excess or hyperbolism are characteristic of adolescence, development breaks down when a hyperbolic frame of mind becomes entrenched or rigidified. Hyperbolic functioning can be enriching to adolescents in trying on vivid or even extreme senses of the self if they have some fluidity.

## Children

Play is the language of childhood, meaning the forms of analysis with children are more fluid than those with adults. Play is a physical and verbal expression of emotions responded to in a liquid – sometimes physical, sometimes verbal manner. The experience of riding the wave of play is as important as the interpretations that eventually emerge from this experience. The shapes and the rhythms of the play have their own vitality. Is there a crash, or do we glide together? Is the ride bumpy and wild or mild and rhythmic?

Playing places both the psychoanalyst and the child in the moment at which things begin to take shape, exemplified in Winnicott's Squiggle drawings. In child analysis, it is often "action that guides thought" (Molinari, 2017, 7). As a child turns my office into chaos, I may have little room for organized thought, but being immersed in action yields to reflection later as I filter through my experiences of a chaotic or sensual scene. I agree with Molinari that child analysis "can refine the analyst's sensitivity to forms of expression other than words" (2017, 4) and "induces in the therapist a more intense sensitivity to rhythmic and formal features" (20).

We also surf by entering a world with a child and letting things emerge. We do this with all patients, but I would argue we do it more so with children – who often enter treatment at someone else's behest. Nine-year-old 'Amy' was referred to me by her neuropsychologist following her diagnosis of Attention Deficit Hyperactivity Disorder (ADHD) and anxiety. These diagnoses have seemed accurate to me over time, but they were of limited help in beginning with Amy. What turned out to be salient was that her father conveyed to me that he had things forced on him as a child, and he was aware he had been too forcing on his daughter in relation to food. This helped me to wait, to take my time with Amy's sometimes expressionless face, with her silences, with her irritability. I didn't really know where we were going, and it took months to get to a point where I could make an interpretation. In some sense, the analytic work was born when I *could* make an interpretation – when Amy allowed me to make connections that could be useful to her. But, in other ways, the analysis started from the beginning, with my uncertainty regarding what we were doing, other than a strong feeling that I should not force or push this child. It was helpful that she seemed to want to come for our time together. At first, she made it clear she did not see why my understanding her would be useful to her, but over time she became much more open.

In a recent session, I could see I caught Amy's attention with some links that I made. As we exited my consulting room, Amy turned back to gaze at me. The experience I had was of Amy loving me and wanting to take me in. It would not be hard to reflect here about positive transference or the early infant gaze at the mother. But what I noticed was a slight hitch in myself – of some hesitation to be loved, I hope not imparted to her. Since that moment, I have been letting in what that gaze meant. This girl (with a moderate level of problems) has allowed a process of great potential. What may have been central was allowing an experience to unfold for her and allowing myself to spend a great deal of time in uncharted waters, not making premature definitions. I am trying to take in this new wave of her love for me. This is not thinking under fire, at least not in the way Bion meant it. Is love such a thing? Is it sometimes hard to fathom love when we don't quite expect it? Perhaps my surfing metaphor is closer here – accepting the beauty of Amy's gaze. Love that is free, free to be given, free to be received – free like the beauty of the ocean and the sky.

## Surfing and the Mobile Frame of Treatment

Child and adolescent analysts surf in relation to ascertaining the location of the problem and with whom the work can be done. Any child analyst will recognize that when presented with a problem in a child, the center of concern may lie elsewhere.

Sometimes the most important work might be done with the parents (see, for example, Molinari, 2022 and Brady, Chapter Two, this Volume). In this regard, I have found Bion's (1961) conceptions of unconscious group functioning extremely helpful in shifting my perspective on the location of the problem in an individual and in a family (Brady, 2011).

Mobility applies to aspects of the frame and timing particularly when working with children. Adolescents are notoriously difficult to set up a regular treatment schedule with. Sometimes, I allow this to play out to see if they can catch the wave of interest in a unique kind of conversation. But, there are many particulars here when a dismissal of the analyst needs to be confronted or creatively engaged with (see Chapter Three, this volume).

## A Child Analyst Surfs with Theory

At best, theory helps us to think in ways we might not have been able to. At worst, it constrains us. Early in my training, a small patient asked me to tie her shoes at the end of the session. She was too little to tie them herself. I hesitated, given the psychoanalytic theory I was learning – don't we interpret instead of act? Retrospectively, this concern is that of a worried beginner – a request trustingly asked disrupts nothing in one's capacity to grasp unconscious material. In fact, the request put me in touch with the developmental level of this little girl. I was hesitant to use theory gracefully at that time – like a beginning surfer not yet able to use a board skillfully.

I was amused when a surfer friend spoke of the hierarchy of surfers in his Santa Cruz community. Likewise, no one has ever said psychoanalytic institutions are lacking in hierarchy. But I imagine that for a surfer riding a wave, like a clinician in an hour, the hierarchies slip away to yield live experiences in the absorption of the moment.

Sometimes, surfing in writing means the effort to follow an idea or an inspiration. Psychoanalytic essays are a form of creative writing using form and language, while the content is clinical and scientific. Sometimes, psychoanalytic writing is collaborative, as is the case of three co-authored chapters in this book. We could say all writing is co-inspired – by our patients, our teachers, our students.

The movement in and out of film, art, literature and psychoanalysis is another form of surfing. I have co-led a film group for psychoanalysts with a film scholar for ten years., through which I have deeply appreciated the complex psychological truths some great directors can convey. Chapter Eight is the creative output of four analysts surfing together on the great Spanish film *Cria Cuervos* by the director Carlos Saura.

## Chapters

The things we struggle with most deeply make us the analysts we are. In Chapter One, I include some personal reflections on work with adolescents. Including the personal in a psychoanalytic book or paper causes an allergic reaction in some, while for others, it is remiss to elide one's characteristics – race, social class, gender identity, etc. as if they could be irrelevant to any clinical encounter. In this chapter, I relate an experience of not knowing. The tolerance for negative capability (Bion, 1970) always seems so much easier in retrospect. In this chapter, I discuss something that eventually became clear to me – not an 'aha moment,' but the mists parting and something coming into focus. I suggest that adolescence can bring unique opportunities for transformation of the adolescent, but also *of the analyst* in preventing our calcification through contact with their developmental vitality.

The second chapter entails my experiencing 'trickiness' from my little girl patient – eventually understood as her way of elaborating on the lying and hiding of an alcoholic parent. The third chapter exemplifies a breakdown in the mobility needed for development. This teen's sense of the uselessness of another's mind left her 'in a hole with a shovel instead of a rope.' Her belief in the obliviousness of her object needed to come to life between us., in order to be understood.

What of the contemporary surfing of gender identity? Teens ride the waves of biological and cultural forces in their own developing sense of self. The sense of self is never stationary, including that of a gendered self. In the fourth chapter, Elena Molinari and I discuss the gendered self of a teen, experimented with by evoking experiences of gender in the analyst

In the fifth chapter, I return to another situation in which surfing breaks down. The anorexic patient epitomizes fear of movement and change. I take up an unconscious adolescent fear of eating up the mother by one's own development. – an extreme form of a central adolescent problem. As Winnicott says, "[G]rowing up means taking the parent's place. *It really does.* In the unconscious fantasy, growing up is inherently an aggressive act" (1971, 144).

In Chapter Six, we will watch a child move towards and away from emotional truth related to a complex origin story. This chapter brings in the complex relationship between treatment and scientific discoveries involving in-vitro fertilization. My co-authors and I discuss an application of Bion's conceptualization of thinking and non-thinking states (K and –K links) to the treatment of a 9-year-old girl.

In Chapter Seven, the surfing is in and out of play spaces, which, for this small boy, collapses into perseverative spaces or nightmare spaces. I refer to Parsons' (2000) view, which states that 'waiting properly' is the necessary state of mind for the analyst. Waiting properly requires openness to catching the patient's wavelength. I attempt to play with the fluctuating material of my small patient and the psychic states evoked in me by him. I also develop the idea of the need for limits of some perseverative play and the corollary in the analysis of adults.

Chapter Eight describes both the collapse of surfing on a societal and personal level during Spain's Fascist regime and a young girl's recovery from this collapsed state. The enforced silence and rigidity of a totalitarian regime are met by the girl's willingness to apprehend the truth. The final chapter considers the cultural, economic and racial divides that affected how the COVID-19 epidemic differentially affected us all, but particularly adolescents. The necessary isolation of the COVID period left adolescents like surfers locked in a room, deprived of fundamental social and psyche-soma expressions.

## Note

1 Bionian and Winnicottian metapsychologies are, of course, quite different, and a rigorous comparison is beyond the scope of this space, but some of the fundamental differences should be apparent to the reader.

## References

Anderson, R., & Dartington, A. (1998). Introduction. In *Facing it Out: Clinical Perspectives on Adolescent Disturbance*. New York, NY: Routledge.

Augoyard, J. (2023). *Excess and Hyperbole, Figures of Idealization for Today's Adolescents*. International Psychoanalytic Association Meetings, Cartagena, Colombia.

Bion, W.R. (1961). *Experiences in Groups*. London: Tavistock.

Bion, W.R. (1965). *Transformations: Change from Learning to Growth*. London: Heinemann.

Bion, W.R. (1970). *Attention and Interpretation*. New York: Basic Books.

Brady, M.T. (2011). The individual in the group: An application of Bion's group theory to parent work in child analysis and child psychotherapy. *Contemporary Psychoanalysis*, 47, 420–437.

Brady, M.T. (2016). *The Body in Adolescence: Psychic Isolation and Physical Symptoms*. New York, NY: Routledge.

Brady, M.T. (2025). *"Daddy's Head is Broken": The Treatment of Children of Severe Alcoholics*. Oxon: Routledge.

Molinari, E. (2017). *Field Theory in Child and Adolescent Psychoanalysis: Understanding and Reacting to Unexpected Developments*. Oxon: Routledge.

Molinari, E. (2022). Child, parents and psychanalyst: Binocular vision in the erotic field. In M.T. Brady (Ed.), *Braving the Erotic Field in the Psychoanalytic Treatment of Adolescents and Children*. Abingdon & New York, NY: Routledge.

Ogden, T. (2024). Ontological psychoanalysis in clinical practice. *Psychoanalytic Quarterly*, 93, 13–31.

Parsons, M. (2000). *The Dove that Returns, the Dove that Vanishes*. New York: Taylor and Francis, Inc.

Puget, J. (2016). How are we to think about the social bond after Freud? *Research in Psan*, 21(1), 109–116.

Winnicott, D.W. (1971). Contemporary concepts of adolescent development. In *Playing and Reality* (pp. 138–150). London: Tavistock.

Winnicott, D.W. (1975). The anti-social tendency. In *Through Paediatrics to Psychoanalysis* (pp. 306–315). New York: Basic Books. (Original work published 1958.)

Winnicott, D.W. (2007). Struggling through the doldrums. In *Family and Individual Development*. Routledge. (Original work published 1968.)

Winnicott, D.W., & Rodman, F.R. (1987). *The Spontaneous Gesture: Selected Letters of DW Winnicott*. Harvard University Press.

# Chapter 1

# Learning to Surf

## Analyzing Adolescents

One of the deep satisfactions of being and becoming a psychoanalyst is discovering one's proclivities. I could not have told you before I undertook psychoanalytic training that adolescents would become a career-long preoccupation. Ogden (1992) describes our experience as human subjects as 'de-centered.' I did not plan, but I discovered my interest in adolescents. Perhaps I could say adolescents chose me rather than I chose them, but that wouldn't be quite right either.

It is true that I have a measure of tolerance for adolescents' frequently scurrilous behavior. I can't tell you how many times a teen has asked me a variant of: 'Can I leave now?' during a session. At some remove, such a challenge can make me laugh. Of course, in the moment, it isn't always all that funny. Such a provocation often reflects an adolescent's own difficulties tolerating him or herself. Often, I can't know if an adolescent will continue to engage with me, however edgily. I can't know if our relationship can gather up their difficulties or whether it will be insufficient to the dangers at hand. What amuses me when I think of such a moment, though, is the way the teen has thrown me a curve ball. What am I going to do with it? What will they do with how I toss it back? Adolescents act in and act out to get to know themselves, and as their analyst, I am in on the experiment.

What are the unconscious pulls that animate my proclivity for adolescents? Certainly, the rebelliousness or subversiveness (Brady, 2018a) endemic to adolescence rings bells for me. My Irish heritage equips me with a strong identification with the oppressed. Like many Irish Americans, my ancestors came to the U.S. during the Great Hunger (commonly called 'potato famine'), a period of mass starvation and disease in Ireland from 1845 to 1849. Though the potatoes did rot of blight in the fields, the crops and the cream and the butter and the beef all went on ships to London, Liverpool or Glasgow. The problem in Ireland was not a lack of food but the price of it. During the famine (under British colonial rule), about one million in Ireland died and another million emigrated (Ross, 2002).

Growing up Irish Catholic and female in Massachusetts during the pedophilia crisis in the Catholic church also fostered my 'question authority' point of view. I partook of a group unconscious that involved the Irish, the Catholic Church and, of course, my family of origin's version of these larger cultural group unconsciouses. For some time, I understood that these sources contributed to my resonance with

DOI: 10.4324/9781003498810-2

adolescents' skepticism. Yet, I sensed that there was something I did not really understand.

Over time, I came to feel that what fundamentally animated my interest in adolescents was that I had been in some danger of missing the adolescent process myself. And while I fortunately did not entirely miss adolescence at its due time, my near miss has left me with a protective feeling for the adolescent process. Perhaps I can give you some sense of this.

## Fragment

*I endured my early adolescence at Holy Name of Jesus Grammar School – a bare, crucifixed edifice in Chicopee, Massachusetts. Irish Americans peopled our school, Polish Catholics and French Catholics in separate enclaves down the street. The glamour lay with the priests, the robes and the incense. The nuns inhabited an inferior realm. We were not the enfranchised children of the next generation. We took what we got.*

*At home, for a time, I had been my mother's girl – read to, sung to and rocked to sleep. The familiarity of the at-home mother. Father goes to work and deals with the outside world – wearing suits and telling jokes. A paradise of Little Women at home. Girl and woman familiar to each other – neither intended for a larger realm. But the pleasures of this. None of the frantic schedules of children intended for success. We baked buttery cakes filled with custard and shimmering with dark chocolate icing. Betty Crocker was our muse.*

*Then, my female fellowship with my mother changed. Perhaps some unbidden hint of sexuality on my part. No longer the little girl dressed in white for First Communion. I could feel the change by the way my mother washed my hair. Showers were mysteriously viewed as profligate by my parents. My mother washed my hair in the kitchen sink. Somehow, shampooing my hair had lost all pleasure for her and for me. Tenderness evaporated – replaced by a rough scrubbing.*

*When I look back, I see the impossibility of it all. I could not stay in my mother's world of daily mass. I had to fumble into the next phase – bell-bottoms and boys with braces. I can see she felt rejected by me. She complained that I did not attend daily mass, but it was she I was not visiting sufficiently, fatally and disloyally decamping to other worlds.*

*Did I become deformed to my mother when my body disloyally decamped towards breasts and hips? She cried the first day I went to the adult instead of the cozy children's section of the library. Her tears made me feel afraid of the adult library – something sinister must lurk there. There was no stopping a subversive flood of ideas – Feminism! Marxism! Buddhism! Franny and Zooey hidden in my closet. Sexual passages read and reread. Union with my mother was over irrevocably.*

You can see that adolescence seemed dangerous to me. I could have used a guide that I did not have. Accompanying adolescents now speaks to that need. Guide is not exactly the right word, as the job is not exactly to show the adolescent a way, but to imagine with them the ways they will find.

The coin of the realm with adolescents is action and experimentation, as that with children is play and that for adults is primarily speech. Sometimes, teens' actions have a playful quality and sometimes are dire or even suicidal. Sometimes, adolescents can think in a breathtaking way as they face the challenge of so much that is new and unfamiliar.

Over my clinical years, I have gravitated theoretically towards Bionian and Field Theory. I value Bion's concepts of waking dreaming and container/contained, as well as his admonition that the only point of importance in any clinical hour is the unknown. The latter is a bracing idea, as I can yearn for the known in the tumult of the clinical process. Adolescents are all about the unknown. They are fundamentally faced with what they do not yet really know about themselves. When they are honest, they often admit this. One late teen tells me that stepping out of his dorm room is an overwhelming challenge. He feels inundated by the multiplicity of responses he has to those around him and knows these responses signal different and often contradictory aspects of himself. How do you even get out the door when you recognize how little you know yourself as a teenager? As we get older, we may know ourselves a little better and be less frightened of the not yet encountered. Or worse, perhaps we become dulled and inured.

The concept of the psychoanalytic field is based on the Barangers' idea that the neutrality of the analyst is impossible. In the analytic situation, there are two people "unfailingly bound and complementary while the situation lasts and involved in the same dynamic process" (Baranger & Baranger, 2008/1961). Any psychoanalysis involves two subjects in space and time. What underlies this process/structure is a shared unconscious fantasy that is the product of unconscious communication and a joint creation process. Ferro (1999) cites the vitality of the bi-personal field concept in freeing us from the idea that unconscious fantasies are only pertinent to one person. The goal of analytic work from a Field Theory perspective is broadening the shared field through the dream work of each of the subjects.

Field Theory would tell you that it is not all that important to pin down the characters in the field. The confused adolescent is me, and I am them. The prospect of care is a character that speaks to my adolescent self, who is afraid of what she is setting in motion.

Winnicott (1965) calls adolescence one of the most exciting things there is. I think that's right, although I also agree with the Uncle Frank character in the film 'Little Miss Sunshine' who advises his nephew Dwayne (who will only communicate with his family via notepad) not to miss his 'prime suffering years.'

When I was in analytic training, I had the excellent fortune to have three adolescents in analysis with accompanying weekly supervision for some parts of the three analyses. I saw younger children and adults as well. Something about the work with the adolescents was particularly riveting. Each of those three teens feels present with me today, 20 years later. Certainly, they provided huge and compelling challenges. They spurred my interest in eating disorders (Brady, 2015a), adolescent substance abuse (2015b, 2015c) and braving erotic feelings alive between adolescent and analyst (2018b). It feels hard even now though, to fully capture the compelling urgency and immediacy of this work. It would be true to say that it was a privilege to study adolescence in-depth and in statu nascendi. It would be true to say that the capacity for self-destruction in those so young concentrates the mind. It would be true to say that the delicacy of immediate and nascent sexual feelings in the room with someone so young is sobering and enlivening. And, of course, you could say all of these are true.

Bion, whose metabolization of horrific battle experience in WWI (Brown, 2012) led to his theory of alpha function, described that the analyst's task is to be able to 'think under fire.' I could think of numerous instances where this is true. But with adolescents, surfing is a metaphor that comes to mind far more often than 'thinking under fire.' For me, surfing catches the adolescent (or myself in their wake), potentially upended, injured or even killed by waves too tumultuous. Yet surfing also captures the sensual beauty of finding a balance, of the thrill of the ride, of a moment of being fully alive. Adolescents in analysis teach me to surf, surfing with me, as I teach them to surf, surfing with them.

## References

Baranger, M., & Baranger, W. (2008). The analytic situation as a dynamic field. *International Journal of Psychoanalysis*, 89, 795–826. (Original work published 1961.)

Brady, M.T. (2015a). Chapter Two, Invisibility and insubstantiality in an anorexic adolescent: Phenomenology and dynamics. In *The Body in Adolescence: Psychic Isolation and Physical Symptoms*. New York, NY: Routledge.

Brady, M.T. (2015b). Chapter Four, Substance abuse in an adolescent boy: Waking the object. In *The Body in Adolescence: Psychic Isolation and Physical Symptoms*. New York, NY: Routledge.

Brady, M.T. (2015c). Chapter Five, "High up on bar stools": Manic defenses and an oblivious object in a late adolescent. In *The Body in Adolescence: Psychic Isolation and Physical Symptoms*. New York, NY: Routledge.

Brady, M.T. (2018a). Chapter Five, Subversiveness in adolescence. In *Analytic Engagements with Adolescents: Sex, Gender and Subversion*. Abingdon & New York, NY: Routledge.

Brady, M.T. (2018b). Chapter One, Braving the erotic field in the treatment of adolescents. In *Analytic Engagements with Adolescents: Sex, Gender and Subversion*. Abingdon & New York, NY: Routledge.

Brown, L.J. (2012). Bion's discovery of Alpha function: Thinking under fire on the battlefield and in the consulting room. *International Journal of Psychoanalysis*, 93, 1191–1214.

Ferro, A. (1999). *The Bi-Personal Field: Experiences in Child Analysis*. London & New York, NY: Routledge.

Ogden, T.H. (1992). The dialectically constituted/decentred subject of psychoanalysis. 1. The Freudian subject. *The International Journal of Psychoanalysis*, 73, 517–526.

Ross, D. (2002). *Ireland: History of a Nation*. New Lanark: Geddes & Grosset.

Winnicott, D. (1965). *The Maturational Processes and the Facilitating Environment*. New York: International Universities Press.

# Chapter 2

# "Daddy's Head is Broken"

## The Treatment of Children of Severe Alcoholics

This chapter seeks to explore the experiences as well as the treatment of children of severe alcoholics. By severe alcoholics, I mean individuals who have had frequent relapses, numerous residential treatment stays, major impairment in work and personal life and related issues such as DUIs, seizures due to alcohol withdrawal and some alcohol-related organic brain damage.

It is beyond the scope of this chapter to review the psychoanalytic literature on alcoholism (Director, 2002; Dodes, 1990, 1995, 1996, 2002, 2003, 2004, 2005; Khantzian & Albanese, 2008; Ramos, 2004; Sabshin, 1995; Taipale, 2017; Yorke, 2003)[1] but I will note some issues for those interested in further exploration. Dodes (2003) contends that there can be a variety of motivations for addiction, including self-medication, affect regulation, object substitution, etc. He stresses that "[P] atients with addictions run the gamut of mental health" (p. 123).

There are multiple determinants of addiction, including genetic, neurological, gender, social and cultural contributions. Here, I am trying to explicate the complex family relationships of children of severe alcoholics and the internalizations of these relationships, which can be addressed in the treatment of children and in corollary parent work.

Analytic writing on the treatment of children of alcoholics is woefully lacking. A Pep-Web search for 'children of alcoholics' yielded mainly papers relevant to adult children of alcoholics (e.g., Eagle, 2014).[2] It is interesting to speculate on this lack. I wonder if it has to do with the systemic nature of the child's problem. The alcoholic parent frequently requires multiple interventions (detox, rehab, 12-step meetings, neuropsychological testing, etc.). These treatments may or may not be successful and, thus, protection of the child through divorce, custody agreements and supervised visits may be necessary. The systemic nature of the problem may also necessitate that the "co-dependent"[3] parent have their own treatment to grapple with their difficulties in facing the severity of their spouse's problems. All of this work is necessary in addition to the analysis or therapy of the child who has internalized aspects of these systemic difficulties. It may be daunting for analysts to accept treatment or conceptualize cases that include such systemic difficulties.

In this Introduction, I will enumerate several difficulties for the children of severe alcoholics, which I will expand upon through clinical material of a girl,

DOI: 10.4324/9781003498810-3

now 12, who has been in treatment with me for the past two years, as well as brief vignettes of two younger children. It is fair to say that children of serious alcoholics (or other substance use disorders) share features with other children whose parents are "distant, unstable or abusive" (Dodes, personal communication). However, I suggest that it is useful to consider what children of severe alcoholics have in common.

There is doubtless overlap between having an alcoholic parent or, for instance, a bipolar parent, but children of alcoholics have to contend with why a parent actively does something that takes them away from the child. In some sense, these children experience the substance of abuse as a mysterious potion, which their alcoholic parent prefers to them. There is considerable evidence for a genetic aspect to alcoholism (Kendler et al., 2011), as well as cultural, familial, environmental and psychological factors. However, children suffer the confusion of why a parent turns to an addictive substance without the ability to understand the parent's motivations and vulnerabilities. Other illnesses may be somewhat less difficult for children to conceptualize.

Yorke (2003) describes that in addiction, the need for the addictive substance is a major preoccupation:

[T]he addict is prepared to do almost *anything*, including steal and lie, to satisfy his/her craving. There are, necessarily limitations on the lengths to which any given person is prepared to go to achieve this end, but those limits may become increasingly elastic as addiction takes greater hold and internal resistances loosen.

(p. 44)

The 12-year-old girl I will discuss further on experienced her father's lies and his drawing her into his efforts to hide his substance abuse from her mother, thus also potentially subverting her relationship with her mother.

Additionally, alcoholics (along with other substance abusers) expose their children to the specific results of inebriation or withdrawal from alcohol. For instance, two of the three children included here witnessed their parents having seizures as a result of withdrawal from alcohol. Likewise, these children all experienced their alcoholic parent sneaking or hiding a substance. I suggest that the experiential world for the children of alcoholics is different than that of a child of a mentally ill parent who does not abuse alcohol or other substances. Of course, parents who have established sufficient sobriety are in a very different position than parents who are actively abusing substances.

I will discuss the following common experiences of the children of severe alcoholics whom I have treated. The first is the extreme difficulty children experience in understanding addiction, particularly very young children. A second issue is the unconscious struggle to repair the damaged parent and to try to protect that parent from strain. Children can suffer guilt at the often-necessary exclusion of the addicted parent from the household unit. These issues can result in a child's pervasive inhibition of healthy aggression. A third confusing issue is mourning for a parent who is still alive and in some contact, yet severely impaired. Finally, I will describe some aspects of parent work in these situations (collateral to child psychoanalysis or psychotherapy), including the work with the 'co-dependent' parent and the difficult attempts to integrate the alcoholic parent into the treatment during possible periods of sobriety.

I will discuss my work with three children: 'Eleanor,' a 12-year-old girl whom I have treated for two years; 'Amanda,' a 4-year-old whose treatment was interrupted at age 5 and 'George,' whom I have worked with from ages 5 to 6. The children of alcoholics I will discuss here had one functional parent (as well as one severely alcoholic parent), social and economic support and the provision of treatment. The case reports discussed here are composites of children with similar circumstances.

## Incomprehension

Many adult issues are intrinsically difficult for a child to understand. Parental illness, death or divorce, issues related to parental sexuality, such as a transitioning parent or the meanings of assisted reproduction (Brady et al., 2019), as well as parental addiction all come to mind. The children I discuss here showed extreme difficulty in understanding their alcoholic parents' conditions relative to the child's developmental level. Eleanor's treatment coincided with her having broader cultural references as she developed from 10 to 12, which somewhat added to her grasp of addiction. A 4-year-old's capacity to understand alcoholism is severely limited. Young children are highly reliant on the sober parent's efforts to protect them from the chaos the other parent's behavior creates while the child's understanding of their familial world can grow. All three parental couples divorced during the period in which I treated their children, so all three children also grappled with the meaning of divorce.

The parents of 'George,' age 4, came for a parenting consultation due to George's defiance and mother's concern regarding father's severe alcoholism. Father has had multiple rehab stays, DUIs and diagnosed alcohol-related organic brain damage. Father's participation during the parenting consultation was erratic and disorganized. In the parenting meetings mother and I would think about what was going on inside George and how to talk with him about father's absences (he was currently in a Sober Living Facility) and how to talk to George. When father would occasionally appear for these parent consultations, mother could see that father was not at all able to acknowledge the problems he had in any way that could be acknowledged to George. I told dad, "Kids worry a lot when they don't understand and don't know what is going on with a parent. I know it is scary for you to face the effects of your alcoholism on George, but it's part of being a parent to acknowledge when we have effected a child." Dad responded that he felt that would "poison" his son's feelings for him. I said, "George will love you no matter what, but what will really hurt him is not being allowed to know his dad." Sessions that involved father felt like they were not going anywhere. I referred the parents for couples therapy, which had similar limitations. At this point, I was not sure how bound mother was to this situation. She asked to take a break from the parenting sessions, which father had stopped attending altogether. Meanwhile, mother did some work in Al-Anon and returned to the parenting work, resolved to carry it through on her own. Mother gradually faced that trying to collaborate in parenting was not possible and began to set firmer limits, restricting father from the home and ultimately filing for divorce.

Now age 5 and in therapy for a year, George repeatedly plays a version of hide and seek, during which he instructs me to look for him with my eyes closed, feeling my way around the office, relying on only the slight hints of sound. I see this play as reflecting George's experience of frustration at not being able to see what is going on with his father (he has been away for multiple residential treatment stays and lives in a Sober Living Facility when he has not been ejected for drinking). I generally stay in the play in this scenario, commenting, "How hard it is when I can't see what is going on," or "It seems like forever, and it makes me mad and sad that I can't see what's going on." At times, I link, "Maybe like George feels when he doesn't know what's going on with daddy," but at this point, I feel it is most important to share in and help carry these emotional experiences without leaving the play. In addition to George's father's absences, there are incidents George can literally *see* but is very much psychically in the dark about. George frequently turns off the lights in my office. I comment on how strange and helpless I feel to be left in the dark.

George's mother has tried to talk with George about father's alcoholism. George related that father took him out in a storm without a jacket, which his mother would never have done. George explains to me that this was because "Daddy's head is broken." When I asked what he meant by this, he added, "Daddy's brain doesn't work right; he let me get really cold and wet." While George could see Daddy had problems parenting, he worried about limits being placed on father by mother. For instance, as he took checkers out of the box, he said, "These checkers aren't letting this one in." George was anxious that father could be excluded from the family unit, while mother was faced with never knowing if father would be sober. Mother told me father hid alcohol or other drugs in the house, so even if breathalyzed, he could at any point shift into an altered state. George had seen his father vomiting from alcohol abuse. I commented to him how confusing it is that his father could drink too much alcohol to the point of making himself sick. George had an almost phobic reaction to seeing someone even other than his father vomit. I linked that, "It's upsetting to see anyone vomit, but especially because daddies are supposed to help kids understand things, and when they drink too much and throw up, they are confusing their kids instead."

Of note, Sesame Street has recently addressed the topic of addiction. Sesame Street has introduced a 6-½-year-old bright green furry character named Karli, who is in foster care while her mother is in rehab. A character named Louie explains to Elmo:

Addiction makes people feel like they need a grown-up drink called alcohol or another kind of drug to feel OK. That can make a person act strange, in ways they can't control.

*Elmo replies:*   Will Karli's mommy get better?
*Louie says:*      Well, she's working hard on it. She's taking good care of her body and mind so she can stay healthy and make good choices.

(NPR, 2019)

Sesame Street's willingness to take on such complex issues is laudable. Of course, child therapists have purposes that go beyond acknowledging addiction and providing hope; the child therapist also tries to allow the child's conscious and unconscious experiences of their parents' alcoholism to emerge in the treatment, including the child's anger, disappointment and confusion. I have found it important to note the child's wish for the parent's recovery (as well as sometimes my own wishfulness in the countertransference). I acknowledge gains the alcoholic parent may have made but also how much has been lost or missed by the child because of the parent's impairment. Of course, this is far more possible with older children. In the section on Parent Work further on, I will relate suggestions on how parents can talk to children about alcoholism.

An important direction for future psychoanalytic exploration is the impact on children of the explosion of opioid abuse and the concomitant explosion of foster care placements (Klaman et al., 2017). Such situations often involve far greater deterioration of the child's familial, economic and social fabric than was the case for the three children I am discussing here. Such disorganized situations likely require the provision of services beyond therapy, such as therapeutic pre-schools or day treatment. A therapist can provide an anchor or containing functions in such a storm. A therapist can assist in the emerging narrative of the child's life. This involves letting the internal object representations emerge in the transference and bearing the related emotional experiences within the transference/countertransference, as well as creating the opportunity for the child to have contact with a therapist's mind to help name and understand. I have encouraged an intermittently incarcerated mother to speak with her daughter about her hope for a better future for the daughter than she had been able to attain herself.

## Repair

In working with children of severe alcoholics, I am often reminded of the Kleinian analyst Henri Rey's (1988) observation that patients often are trying to repair

a damaged inner object without which reparation the subject's self cannot function normally and happily. The patient does not know how to do it. He seeks help with regard to those objects without a conscious realization of what he is looking for.

(p. 457)

'Amanda,' age 5, presented as disorganized, regressed and sweet. In therapy for six months, she repeatedly played with a repair truck tasked with fixing innumerable smashed cars. This play alternated with trying to reach a burning building far too high for the ladder on the fire truck to reach. She asked me to leave the repair truck in place in between sessions, seemingly as an emergent rescue or repair could be needed at any moment. Amanda's mother had just returned from a two-month rehab stay. I said to Amanda, "I know your mom has been away, needing repair," Amanda replied, "I don't need a mom." Amanda would repeatedly ask me, "Why?" about almost anything. I said, "Why is a big question you have in your life for why mommy has the problems she has with drinking and why she comes and goes." Amanda said with some humor, "Why is my favorite question." Amanda had previously witnessed mother frequently drunk, as well as having seizures during times mother had withdrawn from alcohol use. Father was by far the more reliable parent, but had trouble setting limits with mother, who was the more dominant personality.

George (referred to previously), age 5, repeatedly examined me with the play medical kit. When I asked, "What seems to be wrong with me?" George said, "You drank something you are allergic to." In other play, George introduced the idea of a "potion, which could make you good or make you bad." He drew a "scary zombie who could be cured by a magic potion." George's mother had explained to George that while having a glass or two of alcohol could be fine and just make a mommy or daddy relaxed, drinking more alcohol could make a person confused and be bad for them.

The "magic potion" both reflects the alcoholic's effort to solve their emotional problems with an addictive substance and the child's wish for a counter-substance to cure the addiction. At age 5, George's wishes for repair were magical and omnipotent. "I am a superhero, and I will find the good potion to make the zombie good." Another time, George puzzled, "Daddy always comes for visits in a taxi" (his license has been revoked due to drink driving). He asked me, "Why can't he drive if he is bigger than mommy?" I replied, "When he drinks too much alcohol, it isn't safe for him to drive, so it is good he takes a taxi." George said, "He is not going to drink ever again so that he will be able to drive." I gently commented, "How much kids wish their parents would stop drinking when they drink too much, and how hard it is when daddies are not the way kids wish they were." I felt helpless and angry that George should have to internalize a father figure who could not be strong enough to face his problems, though father did love George. At this point, George's contacts with his father were supervised visits, so at least mother and the courts were providing a limit to the disturbance George would have to take in at such a young age.

'Eleanor,' who I will discuss at some length further on, was always anxious at the prospect of saying anything to upset her alcoholic father. She seemed to have no inclination to present him with the numerous ways his behavior had hurt or frightened her. Seemingly, she felt he needed to be repaired before she could be helped. Such an effort to psychically repair or prevent imagined further damage to an ill object could be related to a severe inhibition of healthy aggression, as all the child's energy goes to keeping the ill parent psychically afloat and little or none to the pain of their own experience of the parent's alcoholism.

Eleanor's wish to cure her alcoholic father and her inhibition of healthy self-protective aggression also seemed like an identification with her mother's co-dependence. I commented to Eleanor that while her mother spoke up in many situations, with father, mother often felt uncertain and held back. I thought it was important for Eleanor to see where she could be adopting aspects of her mother that would not serve her well. I also would comment along the lines of, "I'm not sure you liked it when I said x" or "You seemed to drift away; maybe it felt like I was talking too much" in order to be clear that conflict was allowed within our relationship. As treatment progressed, Eleanor became more able to speak up with her peers, her mother and myself. She still says very little to her father regarding his massive impact on her well-being (he now seems to have been sober for a year) but allows me to speak to him in collateral meetings regarding the harmful effects on her I perceive. In collateral sessions, I speak with father about his need to convey to Eleanor that he is strong enough to deal with her anger, but this is very much a work in progress. This case will be discussed at some length further on. But in relation to 'repair,' all family members are aware that they worry father will return to drinking and mother and daughter are unsure whether they can accept father's word about it after numerous violations of trust. I speak both with Eleanor as well as with her parents about "how do you start to trust someone again after they have violated your trust?" I contrast Eleanor's experience of mother having a reliable internal process with father's, which she is not sure about. I encourage father to be able to talk with her about what is going on with him, such as if he seems down or distracted, so that Eleanor might begin to see his (hopefully) growing ability to deal with his feelings instead of resorting to drinking. Father has now been in sustained treatment for a year, as well as taking psychiatric medications and being followed by a psychiatrist.

## Mourning

Children of serious alcoholics are faced with the task of mourning a parent who is often still partially present. Psychoanalytic treatment is aimed at helping children to gain a greater tolerance for painful feelings. Analysts are well aware of the intimate relationship between tolerance for sad affects and the capacity to face reality (Wolfenstein, 1966). Wolfenstein (1966) convincingly discusses the "developmental unreadiness" (p. 97) all children face in mourning a lost parent before the process of adolescence is completed, during which period the adolescent is confronted with the more permanent loss of the parent as a fantasized love object.

Children of serious alcoholics have this normal "developmental unreadiness" in mourning the (partial) loss of their parent due to the parent's failures in being there for the child in multiple ways. This loss can be felt even more profoundly than the loss that occurs when a parent dies. While it may be very difficult for a child to mourn a parent's death, it may be a great comfort to know that the deceased parent did not want to leave the child. An ill or dying parent may have been able to speak with their child about their love for their child and help prepare the child for their impending death. While Eleanor (whom I will discuss later) has been partly able to face her father's serious problems, it often seemed she was waiting for her father to turn into a more able parent, creating a sense of suspended mourning.

While the three alcoholic parents discussed here expressed love for their children and made temporary or (in one case) sustained efforts at sobriety, all three of the children had the experience at times that their parents' addiction outstripped their love for their children. By comparison, deceased parents may be held in their spouses' minds in a relatively unambivalent manner and thus kept psychically alive in a loving and helpful way for their children. Keeping the other parents' goodwill and love for the child in mind is a much more complex task for the spouse of an alcoholic, as they are confronted with the serious failings of the alcoholic parents.

## Parent Work

There are numerous problems in collateral parent work for a child in treatment when one parent is seriously alcoholic, both with the alcoholic parent and to a lesser degree with the 'co-dependent' parent.

The child analyst is confronted with grave difficulties when attempting to work with an actively alcoholic parent. I have generally found it impossible to work with an actively alcoholic parent until some sobriety is established. Rosenfeld (1960/1966) comments that treating the substance abuser is particularly difficult because the analyst "is confronted with the combination of a mental state and the intoxication and confusion caused by drugs" (p. 128).

Additionally, even for individuals in recovery, some brain functions recover and others show limited or no improvement even after periods of abstinence. Mieke et al. (2014) report no improvement following sobriety in several areas of cognition, including semantic memory, sustained attention, impulsivity, emotional face recognition or planning. I have found therapeutic parent work during the initial period of recovery to potentially be contra-indicated as, at that time, alcoholic parents are not likely to be ready to face their impact on their children. This important work may be best delayed until, hopefully, more significant sobriety is attained. Alcoholic parents can be given encouragement with the idea that the best thing they can do for their children is to focus on their own recovery. That is difficult, however, when (for instance) alcoholic parents insist on negotiating custody decisions regarding their children when they have achieved very limited sobriety and have had multiple relapses.

It is challenging, to say the least, to secure the addicted parent's support for psychological work when the very symptom of alcohol or drug dependence is an avoidance of psychological work. Parents struggling with an addiction are not in a psychological condition to readily assume responsibility for their impact on their child, and yet that harm may be ongoing during periods of addiction or partial recovery. In two of the three families I am considering here (George and Eleanor), the co-dependent parent was able to use his or her own therapy and/or collateral parent work to make a more realistic assessment of the addicted parent and then assume the majority of the parental responsibilities themselves.

The alcoholic parent can become antagonistic to the analyst, seeing the analyst as critical of him or her instead of recognizing that the analyst is trying to marshal adequate, realistic parenting on behalf of the child. The alcoholic parent's guilt and shame at their impact on their child(ren) can lead to rejection of the analyst as a superego figure. The alcoholic parent's guilt may also lead to minimizing the problems of the child, which, in an underlying way, the parent may understand, have been caused by the parent's alcoholism. I emphasize that I am trying to support the alcoholic parent to create the kind of relationship he or she would want with their child. I have attempted to help the alcoholic parents explain why they are gone so often (for instance, to rehab) and to acknowledge their addiction to alcohol. This is difficult, if not impossible, until a period of sobriety is established, as denial is such an important part of an active addiction. However, I explain to the sober parents that it is harder for their children to attach to the (alcoholic) parent if they have no chance at all to understand what is going on inside that parent. The child may feel that the alcoholic parent is able to acknowledge the problem honestly, even if transiently, and that may assist the child in having some belief in that parent's commitment to the child.

As you may recall, Amanda is a 5-year-old girl whose mother was a severe alcoholic who was recently sober when Amanda began working with me. Amanda's mother relapsed again soon after the work began and her father stepped in to assume primary parenting responsibility and support for the treatment. However, when Amanda's mother returned from rehab, she immediately pushed for "equity" in terms of physical custody of her daughter – a push that I saw as serving her needs for legitimacy rather than her daughter's need for stability or even her own need to recover more fully. I commented to mother, "You are skipping over your daughter's experience of how things can fall apart, as well as your own need for support to have a solid sobriety." In the treatment, as I described previously, Amanda played that a repair truck came and took away a damaged car. I saw this play as representing mother's frequent departures after relapse, as well as Amanda's unconscious knowledge of mother's illness, mother's need for repair and Amanda's wish that repair could be accomplished. Soon after Amanda's mother's return from her stay in rehab, she convinced Amanda's father to terminate the therapy. In such situations, the reparation that can occur if the alcoholic parent takes account of their impact on their child is forestalled or perhaps may never happen.

In collateral parent work, I suggest that children worry a lot when they don't know or are uncertain about what is going on with a parent. While I always make an effort to help parents find words to describe addiction, this is a tall order with young children. I invite the alcoholic parent to take on naming their own problem to their child, but this may be impossible or very superficial unless significant sobriety has been established. Words that the sober parent and I have arrived at are: "Mommy/Daddy has an illness that involves drinking too much alcohol" or "We all get anxious, but sometimes people drink too much alcohol to try to feel better, but instead it makes things worse."

The co-dependent parent can request that the analyst set limits on the other parent. In those situations, I try to empathically explore what makes it difficult for that parent to set limits or ultimately divorce the addicted parent. George's co-dependent mother initially thought of families in which there is a divorce as "not being a normal family." Keeping an illusion of normalcy was, at first, of prime importance to her. However, George's mother began to realize that it was impossible to collaborate with George's father, as she saw that his out-of-control drinking, concomitant lying and hiding continued unabated. With my support, George's mother was able to insist on supervised visits for father with their children.

Again, recall Amanda, the 5-year-old with an alcoholic mother. Amanda's co-dependent father frequently asked my advice regarding how he should handle custody and other arrangements with Amanda. I pointed out that he rightly thought I had knowledge about children he might not have. I said that my role was not only to assist him by telling him what I thought good decisions would be but also to help him to know and understand himself and his own family better so that he could make those decisions in a good way himself. In this case, my work with him was only partially successful. When Amanda's mother returned again from rehab and pushed for "equity" in custody arrangements for Amanda, father agreed far too readily, ignoring that Amanda's mother repeatedly and quickly slid back into abusing alcohol.

In the following discussion of Eleanor's treatment, I will make it clear how crucial parent work is in families in which one parent is an alcoholic and how important it is also to address the family group dynamic when a child has a parent who is seriously addicted to alcohol (Brady, 2018).

## Eleanor

'Eleanor' was referred to me at age ten by a substance abuse specialist who had evaluated her father. The specialist described her father as a severe, chronic and relapsing alcoholic. He added that the father "gas-lighted" his wife and daughter when the father started to relapse. The specialist was emphatic about the daughter's need for treatment, as he saw her as being quite depressed. I scheduled an initial appointment with both Eleanor's mother and father. Eleanor's father did not appear for the first visit, which I took to be meaningful, as he had at least nominally accepted the recommendation for his daughter's treatment. Mother told me that he had not come to meet with me as he was out drinking because he felt guilty. I made a second attempt to meet with both parents – and for that appointment, father did appear, looking extremely shaky, as if he were both quite nervous and withdrawing from alcohol.

Mother described Eleanor as very bright and verbal but acknowledged that she seemed sad.

During my initial appointment with Eleanor, we had the following exchange:

*A:* Your mom and dad told me that dad has an alcohol problem. I'm sure you've noticed. I'd want you to be able to talk about it.
*E:* My dad took me to a restaurant to get lunch, but then he ordered a lot of drinks and told me not to tell my mom. And once, we went to the drug store, and he had to stop and sit on the floor.

Eleanor and I came to describe father's behavior in the drug store incident as his being "tricky." I was concerned that he was involving Eleanor in his drinking and putting her in a bad situation in relation to her mother by asking Eleanor to hide his drinking. Additionally, Eleanor had to feel guilty at noticing the obvious. I supported the mother in thinking of her daughter first and recommended that Eleanor not spend time with her father while he was drinking and that she not spend substantial time with him until he had established some period of sobriety. Mother told me that when she brought up to father the possibility of his moving out, he had said she was "taking my daughter away." Soon after my initial evaluation, Eleanor's father left home, and her mother told me, "He is holed up somewhere drinking himself to death." Mother accepted my recommendation of a twice-weekly treatment for Eleanor.

Periodically, Eleanor's father would reappear. I helped her mother set limits as I was concerned that Eleanor's childhood could be in a chronic crisis. Eleanor was experiencing insomnia and nightmares, particularly of "zombies who are not who they say they are." She was afraid to sleep without her mother. Themes of disappointment, anger at feeling deceived and having "bad luck" emerged in my early work with her. I commented, "It is confusing that you love your dad and he loves you, even though he is not being a good dad."

Over the months ahead, Eleanor settled into treatment while her father was away, relapsing. Her mood was dysphoric, and she continued to be terrified of zombies. She told me of a dream in which "a zombie ate a kid" and another in which "a house could slide off a cliff." Eleanor did not make any associations to her zombie dreams, but she was receptive to my comments about how confusing it was to have a father who could appear sweet yet did so many things that frightened her.

Several months into Eleanor's treatment, her father entered residential treatment and asked to see Eleanor. I felt that mother agreed to this rather too readily, without establishing any expectations of father. Eleanor and her mother traveled to visit father in his residential treatment program. He left the program Against Medical Advice (A.M.A.) shortly after their visit. When I met with Eleanor's mother, I challenged her for not having paused to think things through with me before choosing to visit father with Eleanor. In this context, Eleanor's mother told me of a child-hood car accident in which both she and her best friend could have died, but she survived and the other child died. I thought that mother was caught in a transfer-ence reenactment with father, playing out loss and survivor guilt. This heretofore unconscious dynamic had undermined her own (otherwise) good judgment.

I felt mother really grasped my interpretation of her unconscious guilt and sub-sequent difficulty protecting herself and Eleanor from father's illness. There were several situations in which she turned to me because she felt my judgment about how to protect Eleanor was better than her own. This demonstrated important insight on mother's part into unconscious interference in her judgment. However, as the treatment went on, I felt that mother often fell back on the defenses of not thinking things through and accepting suffering as an acceptable consequence of survivor guilt. As she put it, she often "put one foot in front of the other" instead of paying real attention to the dynamics in the family, glossing over the pain the father's alcoholism caused and then insufficiently protecting herself and Eleanor.

Eleanor is a poised child who never looks disorganized or intensely upset in sessions. Mother finally confessed to me that she had not wanted to tell me that at home, Eleanor had picked up a knife and threatened to cut herself with it or to drink bleach. At times, Eleanor hit herself at home. I told Eleanor's mother that she needed to tell Eleanor that she (mother) had told me about these terrible upsets or else Eleanor would believe her mother did not feel that Eleanor's painful feelings could be helped. In my next session with Eleanor, she told me that her last upset started when a fountain pen her father had given her was broken. I interpreted that she was intensely sad and angry that her father seemed broken and unable to be a father and that she and her mother were left to deal with the anger at him by themselves, as he wasn't there. I told her she could express anger when she was with me.

Another theme at this point in the treatment was Eleanor's ongoing fear of sleep-ing without her mother. She told me, "I am afraid to wake up and find my mother not there." I said, "You have largely lost one parent and fear losing another." She was now 11 and about a year into treatment. I felt that it was time to address the need for mother and daughter to sleep separately. Eleanor also expressed fear to me that her mother could have a relationship with a new man. I thought that Elea-nor was trying to forestall this eventuality by sleeping with her mother, as well as trying to allay her own intense fears of being alone. I thought that her mother was too afraid of Eleanor's anger. I worked to help her mother gradually insist that Eleanor sleep by herself. This process began with mother staying with Eleanor in Eleanor's room until she fell asleep. There were many ups and downs to helping Eleanor be able to sleep by herself in her own room, but she gradually made pro-gress with mother's encouragement and my interpretations regarding her anxiety at separation.

I felt that it had been correct to advocate for limited contact between Eleanor and her father after he left residential treatment A.M.A. Letting him visit in an unlimited way could expose Eleanor to too much disappointment and sorrow. Elea-nor was very disillusioned and sad during her fifth grade year (which followed this episode). As the academic year went on, she seemed less burdened by depression and anger.

A year and three months into Eleanor's treatment (now towards the end of fifth grade), father was again in touch. He said he had been sober for two months and was now working with a psychiatrist and a substance abuse therapist on an out-patient basis. He expressed regret (in a phone session with me) at having hurt Eleanor and willingness to take current contact slow as "I don't want to hurt her." He offered for me to speak with his therapist, which I did. The therapist said that father was becoming more stable and steady. I told the therapist that the last family reunion had been overly optimistic, as father had left the program A.M.A., soon after the reunion. I expressed sympathy to the therapist and father about the wish that he have more contact with Eleanor but suggested this should be limited until he had a more sustained sobriety. Over the next couple of months, father and daughter started to have daily video chat conversations. I felt that father's attitude was more sincere this time. He expressed, "My goal is to work up to seeing her," indicating that he was assuming more responsibility for necessary repair.

Eleanor's mother is aware of being "co-dependent" with father. Mother said, "I fear rocking the boat." In a joint phone session, she told Eleanor's father, "My worry is that talking about the divorce, as well as talking about how you have hurt Eleanor, will destabilize you. Like you recently made her feel guilty when you said, 'I'm here eating a burger by myself.'" Father was able to respond non-defensively. He said, "I find the distance from her overwhelming, but I know that I'm playing catch-up and I have a deep appreciation for my ignorance."

After a couple of months of near-daily phone contact between Eleanor and her father, Eleanor's mother agreed to a visit for herself and Eleanor with her father, who was in treatment in another part of the country. Mother told me she was tempted just to visit suddenly, without too much notice for the father or Eleanor, as she felt anticipating such visits could lead to downturns for Eleanor. I acknowl-edged her fear but strongly advocated against this, saying that if the visit with Eleanor's father was disappointing, we would need to deal with Eleanor directly about that. Their brief visit went reasonably well, and another was planned for later in the summer. Meanwhile, Eleanor's mother had filed for divorce some months ago and needed her father to sign some papers during this second visit. Again, mother expressed fear and hesitation to face this potential conflict with Eleanor's father. I encouraged mother to approach him in a straightforward man-ner and not to hide it from Eleanor, as Eleanor needed to see her mother being able to face difficulties with her father. Mother did so. I was impressed that during the visit, Eleanor's mother brought up that they had all gotten sad at the end of the prior visit and that this time they could talk about their feelings about saying goodbye beforehand.

As Eleanor prepared to enter sixth grade (a year and eight months into treat-ment), both she and mother expressed the desire for Eleanor to cut back her treat-ment to once a week. I agreed that Eleanor's mood had changed for the better but commented that her improvement had been recent. I recommended that they allow for more time so that her gains could stabilize. I was also aware that while father was progressing, his problems were significant and had the potential to destabilize Eleanor. Both mother and daughter felt that the entrance to middle school would mean that Eleanor had less time, and after a pause, they proceeded to reduce her session frequency to once a week.

Eleanor was anxious starting sixth grade. She reported a nightmare in which "there was a zombie and my mother was saying it was not dangerous." Characteristically, she did not report associations or thoughts about the dream. I commented that: "Part of you may be afraid that by agreeing to reduce our sessions, your mother and I are minimizing fears you have, even though another part of you wants to make this change." Eleanor did acknowledge the possibility that she was minimizing her fears. Fortunately, she gradually adjusted well to sixth grade, and her progress continued. During this time, I recommended to Eleanor's mother and father that if her treatment was to be reduced, it was important that they meet (with me or with a family therapist if they preferred) regularly to discuss how to parent together as their family changes. While they have met with me occasionally, neither parent pursues these meetings in a regular way, revealing both parents' ongoing avoidance of emotional difficulty and conflict.

Eleanor and I began to talk about what it would be like to have father more involved again, though in a different way than when the family had lived together. She told me about a film in which a wife divorces her husband because she considers him unreliable. He, in turn, disguises himself to have more contact with his children. Eleanor seemed to be recognizing that her father could love her but not be a full partner to her mother or to be able to be an equal parent. Both love and loss seemed present in this story. Eleanor also talked about her worries, for example, her fear that father was drinking during the video chats if she saw he had a beverage in his hand. Both mother and daughter struggled to sort out their past experiences of father's drinking and how to read signs of whether or not he was drinking now. He did seem to have made progress, but I myself did not really know how solid his sobriety was.

I will leave my story here, as it is a work in progress. Recently, I asked Eleanor what she hoped for, as her family seemed to be reorganizing in a new way. She told me, "I hope we will be a talking family." I was touched that despite the significant problems Eleanor still faces (given her father's condition), she has gained some sense that a family can face problems. Before becoming a "talking family," the family was lost in feelings that couldn't be put into words.

## Conclusion

I have tried to show the relational and intra-psychic problems children of severe alcoholics can face. Across developmental levels, the children I treated all had severe difficulties in understanding their alcoholic parents' condition, but this was particularly true of the younger children. The children I treated struggled in various ways with the fantasy of repairing their ill parents, and they all attempted to protect the ill parents from their own anger and disappointment. At times, the children's ability to come to terms with the loss or mourning of their parents was put on hold, awaiting the recovery of that parent. Of course, the alcoholic parents might or might not attain sobriety. The ability of even a sober alcoholic parent to understand the impact of their addiction on their child might be quite partial. For instance, Eleanor was relieved at her father's sobriety but then struggled with his unstable moods. His sobriety required him to confront an underlying depression that had contributed to his alcoholism.

I have emphasized the importance of parent work to aid the "co-dependent" parent to protect their child sufficiently. In two of the three cases discussed here (Eleanor and George), the "co-dependent" parent did significant work to understand his or her own contribution to family problems. I will add, in conclusion, that though any alcoholic in recovery would rightly acknowledge the vulnerability to relapse, it has been heartening to see Eleanor's father now sober for a year. Eleanor's family is gradually developing a different way of being together than the one that existed before the crisis of father's worsening alcohol abuse. Such a family might always have a sort of fault line in their sense of stability, but also may also have a meaningful sense of the possibility of recovery and growth.

## Notes

1  I have written elsewhere on substance abuse in adolescence (Brady 2016a, 2016b).
2  With the exception of a paper on mother-infant group psychotherapy (Belt & Punamaki, 2007).
3  Al-Anon recognizes the role of the spouse of an alcoholic as potentially an 'enabler' of addiction. The concept of co-dependence emerged out of the treatment of alcoholics. Spouses can unconsciously support the behavior they are ostensibly trying to control, by protecting the alcoholic from the consequences of his or her actions, e.g., by covering for them, trying to manage them, etc. This can become a shared system of denial and avoidance of the pain of facing difficult choices. The co-dependent partner's focus on their spouse can reveal a tendency to merger and mask a problem with being able to make his or her own decisions and to be able to conceive of a life without the addicted spouse.

## References

Belt, R., & Punamaki, R. (2007). Mother-infant group psychotherapy as an intensive treatment in early interaction among mothers with substance abuse problems. *Journal of Child Psychotherapy*, 33(2), 202–220.
Brady, M.T. (2016a). Chapter Four: Substance abuse in an adolescent boy: Waking the object. In *The Body in Adolescence: Psychic Isolation and Physical Symptoms*. New York, NY: Routledge.
Brady, M.T. (2016b). Chapter Five: High up on bar stools: Manic defences and an oblivious object in a late adolescent. In *The Body in Adolescence: Psychic Isolation and Physical Symptoms*. New York, NY: Routledge.
Brady, M.T. (2018). Chapter Seven: Parent work in adolescent analysis: An application of Bion's group theory. In *Analytic Engagements with Adolescents: Sex, Gender and Subversion*. Abingdon & New York, NY: Routledge.

Brady, M.T., Anzieu-Premmereur, C., & Carey, K. (2019). *Who Am I and How Did I Come to Be? Children with Complex Reproductive Origins.* Symposium, February 9, 2019, American Psychoanalytic Association Meeting, New York, NY.

Director, L. (2002). The value of relational psychoanalysis in the treatment of chronic drug and alcohol use. *Psychoanalytic Dialogues,* 12, 551–579.

Dodes, L. (1990). Addiction, helplessness and narcissistic rage. *The Psychoanalytic Quarterly,* 59, 398–419.

Dodes, L. (1995). Chapter 7: Psychic helplessness and the psychology of addiction. In *The Psychology and Treatment of Addictive Behavior* (pp. 133–145). Madison, CT: International Universities Press.

Dodes, L. (1996). Compulsion and addiction. *Journal of the American Psychoanalytic Association,* 44, 815–835.

Dodes, L. (2002). *The Heart of Addiction.* New York: Harper Collins.

Dodes, L. (2003). Addiction and psychoanalysis. *Canadian Journal of Psychoanalysis,* 11, 123–134.

Dodes, L. (2004). On: What can we learn from psychoanalysis and prospective studies about chemically dependent patients. *The International Journal of Psychoanalysis,* 85(6), 1507–1508.

Dodes, L. (2005). Reply to Dr. Fleming. *The International Journal of Psychoanalysis,* 86(2), 550–551.

Eagle, M.N. (2014). Psychoanalysis needs a better developmental theory – Can new perspectives in biology help? *Neuropsychoanalysis,* 16(1), 29–33.

Kendler, K.S., Gardner, C., & Dick, D.M. (2011). Predicting alcohol consumption in adolescence from alcohol-specific and general externalizing genetic risk factors, key environmental exposures and their interaction. *Psychological Medicine,* 41, 1507–1516. http://dx.doi.org/10.1017/S003329171000190X

Khantzian, E., & Albanese, M. (2008). *Understanding Addiction as Self Medication: Finding Hope Behind the Pain.* Lanham, MD: Rowman and Littlefield.

Klaman, S.L., Isaacs, K., Leopold, A., Perpich, J., Hayahi, S., Vender, J. Campoplano, M., & Jones, H.E. (2017). Treating women who are pregnant and parenting for Opiod Use Disorder and the concurrent care of their infants and children: Literature review to support national guidance. *Journal of Addiction Medicine,* 11(3), 178–190.

Mieke, H.J., Schulte, M., Cousijn, J., den Uyl, T., Goudriaan, A., van den Brink, W., Veltman, D., Schilt, T., & Wiers, R. (2014). Recovery of neurocognitive functions following sustained abstinence after substance dependence and implications for treatment. *Clinical Psychology Review,* 34(7), 531–550.

NPR. (October 11, 2019). *'Sesame Street' Doesn't Shy Away From the Topic of Addiction.* www.npr.org/2019/10/11/769193121/sesame-street-doesnt-shy-away-from-the-topic-of-addiction

Ramos, S.D. (2004). What can we learn from psychoanalysis and prospective studies about chemically dependent patients? *The International Journal of Psychoanalysis,* 85(2), 467–488.

Rey, J.H. (1988). That which patients bring to analysis. *The International Journal of Psychoanalysis,* 69, 457–470.

Rosenfeld, H. (1960/1966). On drug addiction. In *Psychotic States: A Psycho-Analytical Approach* (pp. 128–143). New York: International Universities Press, Inc.

Sabshin, E. (1995). Psychoanalytic studies of addictive behavior: A review. In S. Dowling (Ed.), *The Psychology and Treatment of Addictive Behavior* (pp. 3–15). American Psychoanalytic Association Mongraph 8. Madison, CT: International Universities Press.

Taipale, J. (2017). Controlling the uncontrollable. Self-regulation and the dynamics of addiction. *The Scandinavian Psychoanalytic Review,* 40(1), 29–42.

Wolfenstein, M. (1966). How is mourning possible? *The Psychoanalytic Study of the Child,* 21, 93–123.

Yorke, C. (2003). Commentary on "understanding addictive vulnerability." *Neuropsychoanalysis,* 5, 42–53.

# Chapter 3

# The Oblivious Object

This chapter will consider children with an unconscious relation to an 'oblivious object.' I have spent time considering these issues because they pertain to children (or adults) who tend to find the analyst useless. The conceptualization of an unconscious relationship to a 'stupid object' was introduced by Alvarez (2012). She discusses narcissism or what presents like narcissism in children (children whom she aptly describes as 'not easy to like'). The conceptualization of children with an unconscious relation to an 'oblivious object'[1] is related and presents additional challenges for clinicians to identify and work with. Such children may admire their sometimes highly accomplished parents yet unconsciously experience their object(s) as oblivious to their internal world. The parents I am describing are well in certain respects but chronically unavailable to complex or messy emotions in their children. Conceptualizations of unconscious relationships to stupid or oblivious objects are, of course, relevant in adults as well. But here, I discuss these issues in children as it can be informative to see troubling object relations early in their development.

I will first describe Alvarez's description of a stupid object and some of her ideas regarding narcissism in children. I will then briefly relate Klein's and Bion's theories of unconscious object relations as underpinnings for the consideration of a stupid or an oblivious object. I will next differentiate an 'oblivious' from a 'stupid' object, although such conceptualizations are closely related. I will then provide clinical material of a 13-year-old girl in treatment in order to consider these ideas. I will also describe the somewhat normal developmental tendency for adolescents to consider adults as oblivious.

## The Stupid Object[2]

Alvarez has described a type of internal object that is not exactly felt to be bad but rather stupid and useless. She observed this unconscious object relation in some children of drug addicts, alcoholics or in cases of maternal depression. Such children lay parent dolls on the floor when using the doll house – literally reflecting a sense of no figure to look up to. Alvarez comments that the lack of someone to look up to can lead to cognitive dullness in a child as there is no magnet, no mystery and

DOI: 10.4324/9781003498810-4

insufficient excitement to evoke any curiosity. Such children have no concept of an object who is intelligent – no sense of an adult having an interested and interesting mind. These children see their internal object and potentially adults in general as weak, useless, unprotective and unprotected.

Alvarez's description of 'stupid' objects overlaps with depressed or damaged objects. It may be possible for children to see the limitations in such objects and gradually differentiate them from other adults. When problems in parents (such as drug addiction, alcoholism or depression) are named in the environment, it is easier for children to make differentiations. For instance, I treated a boy from a wealthy family whose mother suffered from depression. His memories of her from his early childhood are all of her being in bed. While he loved her, he certainly saw her as useless. He saw his multiple nannies and other household staff as more emotionally and practically available, but he was never really their primary concern. His sense of his mother's limitations (which, of course, she did not want to suffer), were not denied in the family and could be named. He experienced the depressed aspect of his mother as uninterested, and so, in Alvarez's terms, 'stupid' – not capable of expressing interest in him nor generating interest from him. As Alvarez says, children of such parents do not see the parent as bad but as useless. We could wonder if a 'bad' object could be more animating for a child (than a stupid object), in that the child might feel hate towards their parent instead of indifference. Of course, these distinctions are to aid our thinking and are not absolute. An absent enough object (such as the boy I am referring to) also generates some hatred, albeit towards a weak/'stupid' object.

Alvarez suggests that for therapists, the experience of being with an emotionally deprived child with a stupid, uninteresting object might be similar to being with a devaluing child in that the therapist might experience him/herself as uninteresting. Such distinctions can meaningfully guide therapists in our reflections and interventions.

Alvarez describes subtypes of narcissistic states of mind in children. She differentiates normal self-centeredness from 'pathological' self-centeredness in terms of the normal child's ability to acknowledge nurturing. Alvarez says that the sense of a stupid object may arise in a child with some beginning experience of a lively object but who suffers a narcissistic injury. In Bionian terms, the unmetabolized experience of narcissistic injury is projected into the object – hopefully to occasion emotional work in the parent or analyst. If the narcissistic woundedness is not transformed, a child may develop a more ongoing reliance on contempt. Alvarez notes that a more complacent attitude of contempt can signal the beginning of a more permanent sense of superiority in a child.

## Unconscious Object Relations

Alvarez uses Klein's conceptualization of an internal world organized around central unconscious relationships between aspects of the self and complementary and corresponding objects (Klein, 1975). I am also placing this understanding of unconscious object relations within Bionian (1962) developments regarding container/contained.

The concept of an internal object is not intended to imply an exact representation of a parent but to be influenced by aspects of the object, as well as phantasies of the object also affected by the child's own processes. For instance, an aspect of a parent at a particularly difficult time may be internalized by a child and have an outsize influence on the child. Additionally, children relate to different facets of their object representation at different moments, for instance, at periods of comparative ease or comparative strain.

Klein (1975) saw an infant's earliest development as characterized by primitive phantasies. In her view, the infant's experience of loving caretaking confirms the sense of a good phantasied object or softens the phantasy of a bad object. She saw the primary object of earliest development (the paranoid-schizoid phase) as experienced alternatively as ideal or persecutory due to splitting processes and paranoid anxiety. Splitting allows the infant to make order out of a chaotic experience. A predominance of good over bad experiences is necessary in order to be able to proceed to the next stage, the depressive position. Klein did not view development as based solely on the internalization of good or bad experiences but that an internal predisposition to envy might modify gratifying experiences.

Klein held that the badness or anxiety too difficult to experience inside the self is evacuated out into the other through projective identification. Bion (1962) acknowledged Klein for her insights into projective identification but also took the concept in an expansive, new direction. He saw projective identification as not just a mechanism of defense but as the first mode of communication between mother and infant – as the first rudiment of thinking.

In Bion's view, the infant conveys his fears to his mother[3] by projecting them into her for her to receive and know. The mother hopefully receives the fears and struggles to contain them by giving them meaning. The child's gradual ability to know him or herself is facilitated by being taken in and known in his mother's mind. I consider this a territory where the sense of an 'oblivious object" can develop. Some of the children I am considering have loving parents, but parents who have little idea what to do with a child's complex or difficult emotional experience. This leaves a divided experience for the child, conscious love and admiration for and from the parent(s), but with little hope for anything better than oblivious misattunement.

According to Bion, reverie is the capacity of the primary object to love and think about his or her infant, gradually allowing the infant to internalize a parent who is able to think. The infant can ideally absorb the experience that his or her feelings can be modified, understood and related to. The lack of the experience of reverie leaves the infant without the sense that emotional experiences can be thought about. Sometimes, 'oblivious' parents have some recognition that they do not understand their child (this was the case for the mother of Frances, whom I will describe further on). Such parents don't know what to do with emotion but rather turn to other aspects of themselves or their child – such as an emphasis on academic or athletic success. Some parents avoid any knowledge of their lack of emotional understanding of their children and emphasize their material provision for the child.

Bion saw the personality as constituted by two elements – contained and container – in a dynamic relationship, with the contained continually seeking a container. In an attuned relationship between a mother and baby, a sense of a loving relationship can be internalized into the infant's personality, which transforms into an internal healthy container and contained dynamic in the infant. Alternatively, in a misattuned relationship between a mother and baby, a useless container can be internalized – for example, an obliviousness to one's own experiences. In Bionian terms, oblivious parental containment creates starved emotional content, as well as oblivious internal containment.

The analyst may need to be careful not to reject the projective identification of obliviousness defensively. Tolerating this projection can gradually lead to understanding the child's expectation of obliviousness. Paradoxically, it may be the analyst's willingness to be experienced as oblivious that can allow the child to gradually internalize an object that does not evade the child's experience. On the other hand, the child's disinterest in the analyst may need to be challenged for some sort of breakthrough to a new experience.

## The Oblivious Object

Much has been written (e.g., Mondzrak, 2012) suggesting a contemporary culture of narcissism, abandoning children into narcissistic formations. Societal and parental overvaluation of success and undervaluation of children's inner worlds can be the context for the development of an 'oblivious object.' These children may see their parents as highly intelligent in the external world and even idealize and emulate them, but unconsciously experience their parents as unavailable to their deeper selves. Such parents either do not know what to do with their children's emotional experience or are actively avoidant of any difficult emotions in their children. Unfortunately, children may unconsciously identify with not just their parents' professional success but also their emotional avoidance.

Another variant of this problem is parents who also idealize their children, in part to distance themselves from their children's emotional problems. At times, parents seemingly generously interpret their children's actions as positive when they are, in fact, something else. For instance, 18-year-old Stephen related a memory in which he had been embarrassed by his father questioning a waiter. His father noted how 'kind' his son was to be concerned for the waiter. Children's discomfort with parents drawing attention to themselves is fairly common, especially at ages when the children themselves are particularly self-conscious. So, while a rather ordinary experience, Stephen was feeling critical of his father. Father's idealizing of his son left no room for father to notice criticism and be strong enough to think about it. While Stephen's parents seem comparatively benign, their consistent idealization of their son (including his academic excellence) ignored his multiple difficulties.

This left him feeling both he and his parents were oblivious to any way to recognize and approach his problems. His underlying rage at his parents' obliviousness further separated him from them. Neither he nor they really understood his distance from them, but this distance cut him off from taking in the genuinely good qualities they had to offer. His alienation from them was part of the referring issue. I will give a vignette to convey how his sense of an oblivious or useless object came up in the treatment and how his relationship with an oblivious object also left him oblivious to others.

When Stephen started treatment, he refused regular meetings with me. I decided to go along with this for a time to see if his need to come on his own terms might eventually yield some deeper entry into the work. After some months, I told him I would no longer work on this basis and he was welcome to return if he could see his way to meeting regularly. Several months later, he returned. Over the next year, we met once and then twice weekly, but he missed many sessions without notice. We worked through some of the meanings of these withdrawals, including his fear of his suicidal thoughts and his fear he was mentally ill. Over the next year, he increased from three to four weekly sessions. He attended his sessions steadily.

In this context, we were in a period when Stephen mainly wanted me to let him talk uninterrupted in his sessions. During this particular session, I was comfortable with this implicit arrangement, feeling he needed to play in the presence of an 'environmental mother' (Winnicott, 1965/1958). I was interested in his various riffs throughout the session. As the session drew to an end, I commented, "I think you know I am with you even when I am silent." Stephen responded, "That doesn't seem important; what's important is what I'm talking about." At this point, my heart dropped as I felt I'd allowed him to play out a scene in which he is addicted to his self-importance and my irrelevance. I said, "You experience me as little more than a placeholder. I think we have to deal with how disruptive it feels to you when someone else comes in." Stephen responded, "What do other people give me? I'm being honest. Well, I guess I've gotten laid three times. What do you want from me?"

Stephen was silent for the first half of the next session. I then said, "I got impatient about you pushing me away last session, and you felt attacked." Stephen responded, "Everyone sucks. What's wrong with being an angry person?" I said, "It isn't actually strong to just be aggressive." Stephen said, "There are a lot of things to be critical of. I don't feel much care." I responded, "You're getting too used to pushing people away, and then you can't see what can happen with another person." I said, "You wind up living in a world of one." (He has subsequently come back to this comment several times.)

The next session, Stephen started by reading a passage from a memoir in which the writer describes a psychiatrist's description of her during a breakdown as almost entirely alienated from other humans' feelings. I commented, "That's a scary picture." This period felt like a turning point in our work. I saw Stephen as unable to deal with my or others' positive or negative feelings toward him. His withdrawal seemed to imply a sense of himself at an emotional level as not having anything to offer (while being exceptional intellectually). His parents had been mostly benign but oblivious to how to deal with his difficult feelings. He had radically withdrawn from them. They were concerned about this withdrawal and initiated treatment because of it. However, they were oblivious as to how to step into his anger. Thus, obliviousness occurred at multiple levels here. His sense of an oblivious object created a rage in Stephen, which he felt his object(s) were unable to deal with. Their unwillingness or inability to deal with his anger added to his contempt.

Stephen's assumption of my uselessness had to be confronted so he could begin to face his contempt, as well as the vast insecurity that underlay his endless criticism. I felt that, to some degree, I had to force my way in with Stephen. He would have been content for some time to treat me as useless even though he was using me. His indifference or obliviousness to my experience was parallel to an unconscious parental communication of 'we don't care how you feel as long as you continue to excel and don't disturb our emotional equilibrium.'

I have written elsewhere (Brady, 2015) about a developmentally 'normal' attitude adolescents have toward parents/adults as oblivious. Adolescents often accuse even seemingly attentive parents of being oblivious. I see the experience of obliviousness as a part of the adolescent separation process. Separation processes can leave adolescents feeling cut off both from their real external parents and also from their experience of an inner helpful object. Parents are pushed away and yet needed. Developmentally 'normal' accusations of obliviousness can be exacerbated when there is some real way the parent is checked out or emotionally unavailable.

Next, I will examine the concept of an 'oblivious object' in a 13-year-old girl of an educated and affluent family. This girl was consciously quite idealizing of her successful and affectionate parents. Her sense of the obliviousness of her object needed to arise in our relationship and be understood in the transference-countertransference field. Such work may allow a beginning sense of an object that can be of emotional use to a child.

## 'Frances'

Frances was referred after she told her mother she felt very anxious and "not right in the head." She had told her mother tearfully: "I have a crushing in my head, and I shouldn't be alive."

Frances attends a private school. Her parents described Frances as "good interpersonally – a reluctant leader who is curious and political." Her parents reported a history of depression on both sides of the family. Mother suffered panic attacks in her early twenties and tried therapy but said: "I didn't take to it. I tough things out."

Pregnancy and delivery were normal, and Frances was breast-fed. Mother went back to full-time work when Frances was three months old. Mother told me that Frances "refused to eat from the au pair the first week I went back to work." Father laughingly described this as Frances being "stubborn." I commented: "This seemed far too young for stubbornness, but rather seemed a sign of distress." Mother said: "I did think she was distressed and that, then as now, I would not work if Frances needed me, but that I didn't know what to do." Compared with father, mother had some sense that her infant was emotionally distraught but was unable to use her perception to respond emotionally and practically.

Many near-catastrophic difficulties preceded Frances's younger sister's birth when Frances was 5. Frances "was stand-offish" after her sister's birth. Currently, Frances's 8-year-old sister sleeps in the parent's bed. Mother started a demanding job a year prior to Frances beginning treatment and travels for work intermittently. Frances is anxious and has stomach aches when her mother is away.

## Course of Treatment

My initial impression upon meeting Frances was that she was in a much worse psychological condition than her parents had conveyed. It felt eerie to be with her. She only spoke if I made a comment or asked a question. When Frances did speak, what she said was often gripping. In the first session, Frances told me she felt "in a deep hole, with a shovel instead of a rope." She said in fourth and fifth grade, she had felt "not good, not bad, murky" and in sixth grade, "I felt doomed and unreal." She currently (summer before seventh grade) often feels like "I am watching myself." I had the impression that she was having a dissociative experience of removal from herself. I inquired into her having told her parents, "I shouldn't be alive." She replied, "I don't want to kill myself; I just wish I could evaporate."

I felt concerned in early sessions that Frances could be having a breakdown or entering into a major mental illness. I felt some hope when she came in to the second session and said, "I like your hairstyle." I tried to ask what she meant, but she could not elaborate. I took the comment as some bit of positive feeling towards me. She also said, "I dreamed I had a puppy with me that I held throughout the day." I said, "The puppy may be a part of yourself that you feel some willingness we care for." She seemed to agree but again could not say more. I told Frances's parents that she was significantly depressed and anxious and recommended that she begin a twice-weekly treatment, which they agreed to.

Frances had a planned two weeks away coming up, the first week a family vacation and the second week to a friend's country home, which she had visited before. I asked what it might feel like for us to have a break so soon after starting. She replied, "Lonely, but you could send me a letter." I soon received an urgent message from mother that Frances felt too anxious to go to her friend's house. Her parents agreed for her to stay home. When she came in, Frances said, "I feel depressed and hopeless, like someone turned the lights off." I felt very concerned about Frances's state and suggested to her parents that I see her each day that week, which they agreed to. I told them, "She has hidden some of how bad she has been feeling because she feels she is supposed to perform."

Frances said during that week, "I feel empty, I feel worse and worse until I blank out," and described "suffocating panic." She denied hallucinations or delusions. I said, "It is very important that your parents and I stay close to you when you are feeling like this." I mentioned the possibility of medication to Frances and asked how she felt about it. She said, "I don't care." In a later session, I told Frances, "Medication is no substitute for our feeling close and would not be forever, but it could help you feel better now." I said I was open to hearing whether what she was going through felt like too much for her. Soon after, Frances told me that she did want to start medication. The psychiatrists I normally work with were away on summer vacation, so I sought out someone who could see her. The psychiatrist said Frances had been having "panic-like events" and intense fears with quasi-suicidal thoughts. He said her parents were concerned with the frequency I was seeing Frances (three sessions a week at this point), and that he had agreed with them that it seemed excessive.

While Frances's parents had initially seemed reasonably trusting, their support wavered during this period. They expressed confusion as to how to know we were on the right track. I said I could understand their worry about whether I was giving their daughter the right care but that it was a good sign that she was talking with me. Meanwhile, I dreamed I was on a ship turning upside down, which meant there would be water on every floor of the ship. There would be an air pocket on each floor, but I would be underwater for a time while everything went upside down. I thought my dream reflected my anxiety about Frances but also the faltering support I had. I asked her parents to come in and meet with me to talk about this directly. I said, "When a child feels overwhelmed, it is really important that the adults around them come together." Without an alliance, it would be very hard to work in this situation. During this period, Frances talked at length about a television show which depicts characters who are sucked into a strange, parallel universe.

Meanwhile, Frances started on an anti-depressant, which was clearly helpful. Her crushing, suffocating anxiety decreased.

The parents occasionally canceled my appointments with Frances. I told them Frances needed to see that our appointments were being treated as important. Shortly after this, I came out to the waiting room to collect Frances for her appointment. She was not there, but her mother was. She said Frances was out in the car, not wanting to come in because she was upset about school and wanted to go home. I suggested to mother that I go down and speak with Frances in the car. In the car, I told Frances that it was especially important we be together when she was upset so she could get more used to having emotions when she was with me. Frances was able to come in and have the session. Mother had been able to support the treatment in not acceding to Frances's testing of the solidity of our work. Here, mother was able not to be oblivious to Frances's need for treatment and my need for mother's support. Since this crisis period, our work has been more stable. Frances is still silent unless I start us off. She then speaks in an animated manner. She doesn't like to talk about her anxiety because she feels it will start again.

At the time of the session I will provide, Frances had just reduced to two sessions a week, five months into treatment. My current struggle centers on helping Frances to deal with her difficulties when she is also genuinely feeling better.

Frances is on time and gives me a slight smile as I get her from the waiting room. She picks up her folder of drawings and sits cross-legged on the couch. She starts to color in the shapes of the outlines she made last time. She is silent. I think about whether to let the silence extend. After a few minutes, I say:

*A:* I was thinking it feels like a ritual when you pick up the markers and start to draw. Like, it almost would feel strange to me if you didn't. And maybe me getting us started is another ritual.

*F:* Nods, silent.

*A:* And there's something nice about rituals, as long as they suit how you feel. What would it be like if I didn't start us off?

*F:* I'd probably say something eventually.

*A:* Just to break the silence?

*F:* Yes. Nothing has happened since I was here last, and I don't feel like talking. I'm tired.

Silence

*A:* Tired from?

*F:* I was up until 11:30 Friday night and got up at 9:00 the next morning, and Saturday, I was up until 11:30 again because my parents went to bed, and my sister wanted me to watch Spider-Man with her. She said she'd do my chores if I'd watch it with her.

*A:* That's hysterical. Because she wanted your company?

*F:* Yeah, and there are some parts that are inappropriate, scary for her. And then my mother woke me up at 8:00 a.m. because we were going somewhere. And I went to bed at 9:30 last night, which is pretty normal, but then having to get up to be at school at 8:00 a.m. and felt like I had a sleep shortage from the weekend.

*A:* So, you had a whole backlog of things that you were doing on other people's timing. I know how nice it is for you when it's vacation and you can stay in bed as late as you like.

Silence

*A:* There are things that are important about noticing when you don't feel like talking and when you do. You certainly don't want to feel you have to talk 'just because.'

*F:* Nods.

*A:* But at the same time, I think last summer we realized that you were really feeling bad, in part because it was hard to want to talk about all that was troubling you.

*F:* I think this is different because it's not like I'm feeling really bad.

*A:* That is different.

Silence. (I am feeling irritated – like, 'Why do I have to figure out how to get her to communicate?' I don't feel there's something developing in this silence. Rather, it's a holding pattern, an avoidance pattern, with a bit of, 'you can't make me.')

*A:* I think I could let you be quiet until you felt like talking, but I'm not sure that would be great. One of the things that scared you most was feeling you could not even want to talk to your mother. So, we are trying to find our way . . . on the one hand, you get to not feel like talking, but I think you also don't want me to just leave you with it without figuring out if the silence is going somewhere.

*F:* Yes, my mom was getting me up on Sunday to go shopping. I don't have a bathing suit to go to Barbados.

*A:* Did you want to do that?

*F:* Yes, I just didn't want to get up, but we didn't wind up going until later. You never go shopping and buy just one thing. I was in the dressing room with my mom, and she kept coming out and saying, 'Do you like this hat, do you like these shorts, do you like these sunglasses?' She comes to me for fashion advice. I save her from wearing plaids and stripes or stripes in two different directions.

*A:* That's funny; you kind of sound like the mom. Or do you ask her for advice, too?

*F:* No, how could she give me advice if I'm the one she gets advice from? The only thing she cares about with my clothes is short shorts. She'll say, 'longer.' Short shorts don't look good on me.

*A:* Some people like going shopping for bathing suits, and some people hate it.

*F:* I just don't like trying on clothes. I have, like, three outfits, this one – my uniform – and then jeans and then leggings and then occasionally a dressy dress. I don't really care about fashion; just what I think looks nice. And then my mom buys a thousand things, she's like, 'You need this, sister needs this, dad needs this' and then she says, 'We need to make cookies,' so we got cookie mix. She's my aunt. My aunt is always buying things for everyone. My mother didn't used to be like that, but now she is. I watched a film last night. The book was better than the film, but the film was really good too. I'd seen it before, but I noticed something I didn't the first time.


*A:* What was that?

*F:* So, the book is narrated by Death. Death knows when everyone will die, so it will say things like: 'It's not his time yet.' This town is getting bombed, and so everyone is going into some shelter basement. And one family is hiding this Jew in their basement.

*A:* Where is it set?

*F:* In Germany, outside of Berlin. And so, when everyone else in the town goes to this shelter, the Jew can come out, and it's the only time he's been able to see the sky for a long time. That seems like it would be worse than death. The narrator, of course, isn't really Death; it's the author's idea of death. There's one point where the main character's street is bombed, and the name of her street is the German word for heaven. So, they are bombing heaven.

*A:* And I guess it would be us bombing heaven.

*F:* Yes, or the British. I wonder whether the author thought of the street as heaven first and then bombing it or the other way around.

*A:* It's interesting. Lots of time when we're reading, we're in the story, but not so much thinking of the author, but you're wondering how the author imagined the story.

We've got to stop.

She puts her drawing in her folder and smiles happily.

### Discussion

During the majority of the hour, Frances does not seem to feel there is any point in talking to me. I think at this point of the treatment, she feels safer seeing me as she has some sense that I have helped to steer her out of deep waters, but I think it is difficult for her to really feel I could be of any help to her. Despite her seeing little use in talking to me, my comment that she had been left too alone with her emotional life may have reached her and she begins to communicate.

We hear of family experiences when her sister and then her mother want something from her (fashion advice). She expresses comparative indifference to these endeavors and seems to feel some superiority over her mother. Then, things deepen with her thoughts about the film. Though it is jarring that she refers to a character as 'the Jew,' she seems to identify with what it would be like to be shut in and not see the sky. This reminded me of Frances's fear of being trapped inside the hole with a shovel instead of a rope.

Frances's preoccupation with death brought to my mind her mother's medical issues before Frances's sister's birth. At one level, Frances is struggling with profound issues of death, violence, heaven and hell. At another level, she is rather vacant and feels no one is up to accompanying her. Her parents and I are seen as useless, oblivious objects. A hateful object in some way would be more activating, while Frances seems to view her objects as harmless and good but as easy to be superior to. When her objects are useless, she is left alone.

### Conclusion

I have found Alvarez's discussion of the stupid object helpful in understanding some children who have little hope of an adult being interesting or interested. I have tried to describe a related concept of children with an oblivious object. It may be difficult for therapists to see how truly oblivious some children may consider adults to be when the child has a conscious attitude of admiration or even idealization toward his/her parents. When children are in the midst of so much activity and their parents are materially helpful, it can be hard to grasp how alone they are with their emotional problems. Frances's parents were forced to seek psychological help for their daughter due to her level of distress, which they still minimized. Some genuine work took place, and Frances was on much more solid ground when she ended treatment a year and a half later. I tried to leave Frances with some sense of the importance of her internal life. However, I felt there was a formidable family defense in the direction of activity and success and little sustained parental access to their own internal processes. Frances had made real progress, but in some ways, I felt that the status quo had been restored.

As we ended, I let Frances know that she had done some hard work to recover her sense of her own individual importance and a deeper understanding of her thoughts and feelings. I am left with the concern that the lessons of this period of Frances's life might feel tempting to forget. A parental need for obliviousness to emotional pain can create children who are oblivious to their own internal worlds. These children's obliviousness is both an identification with their parents and an avoidance of pain that would be required to see their parents' cut-off obliviousness. Such children can look okay until they can't anymore.

## Notes

1 Elsewhere, I have utilized H. Rosenfeld's (1960) conceptualization of identification with an ill or dead object (Brady, 2016). Green (1983) described a mother still alive but emotionally unavailable to a child due to sudden depression caused by severe loss. The parents I am describing here are alive and well in certain respects but chronically unavailable to complex or messy emotions in their children.
2 This section is based on Alvarez's (2012) chapter.
3 Bion uses 'mother' to refer to the infant's primary object; it could equally be a father.

## References

Alvarez, A. (2012). Issues of narcissism, self-worth and the relation to the stupid object: Devalued or unvalued? In *The Thinking Heart: Three Levels of Psychoanalytic Therapy with Disturbed Children.* Hove & New York, NY: Routledge.

Bion, W.R. (1962). *Learning from Experience.* London: Karnac.

Brady, M.T. (2015). High up on bar stools: Manic defences and an oblivious object in a late adolescent. *Journal of Child Psychotherapy*, 41(1), 52–72.

Brady, M.T. (2016). Substance abuse in an adolescent boy: Waking the object. *Contemporary Psychoanalysis*, 52(2), 201–223.

Green, A. (1986). The dead mother. In A. Green (Ed.), *On Private Madness.* Madison, CT: International Universities Press. (Original work published 1983.)

Klein, M. (1975). Notes on some schizoid mechanisms. In *Envy and Gratitude.* London: The Hogarth Press. (Original work published 1946.)

Mondzrak, V. (2012). Reflections on psychoanalytic technique with adolescents today: Pseudo-pseudomaturity. *International Journal of Psycho-Analysis*, 93(3), 649–666.

Rosenfeld, H. (1966). On drug addiction. In *Psychotic States: A Psycho-Analytical Approach* (pp. 128–143). New York: International Universities Press, Inc. (Original work published 1960.)

Winnicott, D.W. (1965/1958). *The Capacity to Be Alone, The Maturational Processes and the Facilitating Environment* (pp. 29–36). New York: IUP.

Chapter 4

# Adolescent Feminine Subjectivities Elaborated via Transitory Objects in the Analytic Field

*With Elena Molinari*

## Introduction

In this chapter, we seek to explore Winnicott's (1966) concepts of the 'masculine' and the 'feminine' within the early mother-infant relationship to explicate how the masculine/feminine dimensions reappear in adolescence. Adolescence is a crossroad between the redefinition of the self and the cultures of the family and society. We will also use Bion's concept of container/contained to examine the group dynamic of family and society that imagines the individual adolescent. The individual interrelates with the shared group unconscious (Bion, 1961) and forms contexts of expectations and norms. We also introduce the concept of 'transitory objects' (discussed later in this section) as a way to capture and track shifting expressions of the masculine/feminine themes of an adolescent girl in analysis.

Winnicott uses the concepts of 'masculine' and 'feminine' not to describe the beginnings of gender and sexuality but to describe the somatic relationship between mother and baby. He terms the 'feminine element' as the earliest relationship between mother and baby before the relationship with the object develops. The feminine correlates with 'being,' not excluding variation but otherness, and basically guarantees continuity of the internal and external environment. The 'masculine element,' on the other hand, has to do with an active relationship with the other and serves to recognize and accept differences. These elements have no relationship to gender; rather, they set up the paradox of relationality in their difference and, if not impeded, become a root of creativity. Winnicott (1966) described the relationship between masculine and feminine as two distinctive but intimately connected elements, just as twins during gestation, though separate and different, brush against each other and lean on each other.

In this theoretical frame, the role of primary aggression is involved in the dynamic of recognizing the *me* and the *not-me*. In order for the object to be utilized and transformed from a subjective object into a true relational object, it must be able to be possessed, to be destroyed by the baby's innate aggression and then to be re-created by him or her. This re-appropriation through aggression, in which the object survives, forms the basis of the capacity to be in a relationship. Winnicott describes aggression as a basic element of psychic function from the origins of life

DOI: 10.4324/9781003498810-5

through the concepts of 'masculine' and 'feminine.' Aggression can play a positive, organizing role during development or, if characterized as a pathological element, can produce relational difficulties.

While Winnicott utilizes the concept of masculine/feminine to describe the first steps of the mind in its impact on the world, Bion looks at the same relational dynamic and utilizes the conceptual tool of the container/contained (♀ ♂) relationship. Bion describes the mouth/breast relationship and the psychic meeting between the mother's mind and the baby's mind through projective identification (Bion, 1962, 1970). He focuses on the need for help from another mind to work through the negative feelings that emerge from frustration. The capacity to learn from experience is highly dependent on the availability of the container/maternal mind to accept projections. If this happens, the baby gradually internalizes the capacity to contain his own mental states.

Bion also utilized the concept (♀ ♂) at a greater level of abstraction, applying it to the relationship between the subject and the group, whether familial or social (Brady, 2018; Obholzer, 1996; Grotstein, 2011). At whatever level it is considered, the relationship of container/contained describes a dialectic essential to subjectivization. Bion's interest is not so much in gendered sexuality as in the mental relationship between container/contained. However, he termed the relationship between container/contained 'intercourse,' thus maintaining its bodily roots. We will, therefore, use this concept as a tool that encompasses many levels of the relationship between minds: the initial level of the relationship with the caregiver, the adolescent level in which the relationship takes on a more gendered meaning and the level with the social group. The culture influences every stage of development with particularities that we will try to highlight. For example, cultural imperatives give a 'sexualized/gendered' meaning even during pregnancy through the parents' fantasies or projections of the fetus. Moreover, in early development, masculine and feminine, as psychic states in the infant, start to take on a more gendered meaning. This occurs as a child differentiates her/himself from the mother, which drives development toward a sense of self, necessarily influenced by others and culture. The inner fantasies of the mother and her ideas about what is acceptable vis-à-vis gender become more conditioned. The child ventures into a word that 'tells' her/him what a proper way is of being in a relationship with gender.

The influence of gender identity intensifies in early adolescence as both internal and external demands require adjustment to changing circumstances. Adolescence is a liminal period when adolescents, their families and their psychoanalysts imagine the unfolding feminine/masculine theme. At this moment, not only is the familial private culture about gender important, but also the social one. As analysts, we cannot lose the concept of a subject that will organize experiences of biology and culture in a unique and not pre-determined form. In psychoanalysis, preconceptions about ourselves, including those related to gender, are examined, and potentially reimagined, by both patient and analyst. The treatment of an adolescent is a watershed moment in grappling with one's sexuality and gender. The tension between the culture-bound and the potential for new imaginings of gender may be an explicit or implicit theme of the work.

Adolescent sexual relationships co-construct and constitute versions of the feminine and the masculine. Such narratives of gender are compromise formations, which include over-determined normativities and yet are idiographic and embodied. Adolescents can ape cultural forms and yet simultaneously 'try on' their own experiences. Conformity to cultural expectations leads to comprehensibility but threatens the unique and the personal. Boundaries of the 'approved' have moved so significantly in contemporary culture that we constantly reimagine gender.

We will relate clinical material from a 14-year-old girl who came into treatment because her mother considered her behavior towards her twin brother too aggressive. The family culture brought expectations about the behavior of a young girl to the therapy. The presenting issue of the relationship between sister and brother introduced the male-female theme into the analysis, which was then present in the analytic relationship at different levels:

- inside the subject in the first stage of development in Winnicott's sense
- in the interpersonal relationship
- as a dream function

The last point refers to Bion's theory about the need for the analyst to consider the analytical relationship as a co-created dream during the session. Masculine and feminine can be understood as a dreamlike composition of different parts of the self and the other.

We will use this clinical material to examine how culture, family and psyche interweave in experiences of gender. We will present an ongoing series of clinical moments between an adolescent girl and her female analyst and suggest that culture-bound experiences of the feminine are subtly reimagined in these moments.

Through the clinical material, we will also introduce the concept of 'transitory objects.' We use this term to describe art produced in the treatment by the analyst and the patient together, similar to Winnicott's squiggle technique. Transitory objects are relational tools able to promote the transition from self-disconnection to connectedness. They have two sides: one that shows internal integration and a second that shows relational change. As Winnicott's squiggle, transitory objects condense within themselves the working-through of a process. In the current clinical work, they were used as a way to capture and track shifting expressions of the masculine/feminine themes of an early adolescent girl.

Child/adolescent analysis informs adult analysis through its emphasis on shapes and forms, which yield the beginnings of representability. This adolescent girl used artistic modalities to create visual representations that convey her emerging grasp of a complex unconscious masculine/feminine situation.[1] Play with a child or artwork with an adolescent can gather unprocessed beta elements into dream/alpha elements, allowing the digestion of complex emotions. We will describe a series of images that gave meaning to previously unthinkable emotions related to the feminine/masculine theme.

Winnicott contends that playing (or, here, artwork with an early adolescent) places both the psychoanalyst and the child in the moment at which things begin to take shape. This is synchronous with Bion's advice that the analyst: "abandons memory and desire (in order to be optimally intuitive and receptive to his own unconscious vis-à-vis the analysand)" (Bion, 1967 p. 136). Reflection and interpretation can occur after a period of the development of play/art experiences.

The conception of transitory objects is also informed by the Baranger and Baranger (2008/1961)[2] assertion that the analyst's neutrality is impossible and that the patient and analyst are bound in a dynamic and complementary bi-personal field, a spatial and temporal structure with its own laws and dynamics, resulting from the joint creation of an underlying shared unconscious fantasy. What underlies this structure is a shared unconscious fantasy that is the product of unconscious communication and a joint creation process.

## Violet[3]

Violet entered therapy at 14 because her mother felt that she was inexplicably overly aggressive toward her twin brother, in contrast to an equally excessive timidity and withdrawal in relation to others. The father, a silent and shy man, said that Violet looked like him and did not share his wife's concerns.

Violet's twin brother did not seem to live up to their mother's expectations and was not very responsive to their mother's solicitations. As a younger child, Violet had been at an advantage in satisfying her mother's needs. She maintained maternal approval until early adolescence as a good student and well-behaved. However, when Violet showed more open anger toward her brother at the beginning of adolescence (even though it was not much beyond a normal level of conflict between adolescent siblings), mother perceived her as intolerably aggressive. The mother was likely projecting a split part of her own unconscious hatred towards her disappointing male child. The mother's difficulty in taking care of two children (not only in a concrete manner) may be shown by the fact that a nanny still lived with the family even now that the twins were mid-adolescent.

I will describe the first two years of her twice-weekly treatment.

My meetings with Violet always took place in the room used for therapy with children and adolescents, a larger one than the room where I work with adults and with a table for playing or drawing. Since the entryway accesses both therapy rooms (which are on opposite sides), if the doors are not properly closed, whoever enters can easily glance into one or the other room. Soon after our meetings began, Violet asked me if she could look at the room that she glimpsed on entering – where, she said, 'We never go in.'

I acquiesced, and we sat on the chairs there for some minutes, close to each other. She observed a series of little paintings on slabs of solidified limestone, which I had done during my analysis. The paintings represented women who, in all probability, embodied parts of myself that were in transformation. For some years, I had kept them concealed, like products of a relationship that was too intimate to be shown, but eventually, it seemed to me that they were entitled to a place that represented an ideal continuity between the room where I had done analysis as a patient and the new one where I practiced as an analyst.

Violet's attention was attracted by two of my paintings: 'This woman seems lonely,' she said to me. Then, fixing her gaze on another painting, she said: 'This one, in contrast, seems to be a ballerina, like me.' Then she added, 'in a trap.'

Her remarks had the effect of arousing in me a cluster of memories, reflections and emotions that seemed not to have been tamed much either in my analysis or in the paintings. Although it may seem absurd, I had never really thought about how my not having been able to pursue dancing (for various reasons that were difficult to accept) had become merged with the tunic with which I had dressed the 'imprisoned' woman. The 'imprisoned' ballerina was thus an image of my very early feeling of not being able to move or to rebel.

The other painting, the only one on a different mounting, represents an adult woman, nude, curled up tightly as though contained in a uterine sphere. Geometric, angular forms take up half the oval stone on which it is painted, in stark contrast to the other elements that resemble a biological setting. To be in contact with the angular parts of one's own mother or of one's analyst, and to be trapped, now appeared to me as elements of relating to each other with a new rapport. When we returned to our usual room, Violet wanted to begin to paint, using some plastic materials.

The artistic objects that marked the stages of our journey – I consider 'transitory objects,' (discussed later on): are objects created by Violet and by me.

I will present the work with this young girl in three segments.

### Doors: Transition and Borders of Setting

My association with Violet's wish to go into a forbidden room – or to open a closed door – was to the doors implemented by Kounellis in Sarajevo right after the end of the conflict in the former Yugoslavia. These doors were filled in with various concrete materials that completely obstructed transit: books, bells, sacks, etc. These materials transformed doors from architectural elements indicating passage to elements that enclose and entrap, becoming symbolic of what conflict can produce: a reduction of tri-dimensionality to life in a flat and potentially lethal space.

My decision to allow Violet to enter the adult room was a response to her desire to enter a 'new place,' as in a different relationship with me. The memory of Jannis Kounellis' exposition pushed me not to obstruct the possibility of development with theory and a rigid application of the setting.[4] I was aware that the frustration of Violet's desire would allow a limit and anger about frustration with the possibility of transforming emotions with words as usual in the therapeutic setting. However, current developments in the psychotherapeutic treatment of adolescents suggest that the setting may be used in a more flexible way as a therapeutic factor given the adolescent desire to change the setting in relation to their development (Laor, 2007; Anagnostaki et al., 2017; Ferro, 2018). Although adolescents need containment that gives them a sense of solidity and continuity, they also need a 'tailor-made' setting rather than the application of anonymous rules. Transforming the setting into a shared space allows the teenager to feel not only involved but co-responsible. Adolescents don't like to feel as passive subjects of an investigation showing their weaknesses and pathology but as subjects whose therapy offers the opportunity to transform difficulties into a demanding self-exploration.

Violet asked me for stones like the ones I had painted on to continue to share and explore this new place we had entered. Not having any at our disposal, we decided to spread some little wooden tables with soft dough made of sand and glue in order to create a surface similar to the backing of my paintings.

Over the course of several sessions, these little tables came to be carved into and scratched with various tools without the end result of any particular representation. In engaging in this project, Violet displayed a mixture of courage and inhibition: she felt able to transmit her rage through this activity. At the same time, it frightened her to a degree that she continually asked for confirmation that what she was doing was right. My approval was indispensable in her discovering her capacity to express her feelings in this external form, but my refraining from giving advice, as usual in the analytical setting, also allowed Violet to be pleasurably surprised by her results. This work, together with non-symbolic signs, was similar to the squiggle play of Winnicott, a way to be in a relationship able to introduce the experience of reciprocity: "me a little and you a little" (Winnicott, 1959; Stefana & Gamba, 2018).

So, we decided to color the tables, and once they were dry, put water on them to remove any excess and create a more variegated effect. The result was one of surprising beauty: the aggressive action now represented something rising up, far from the stereotype of destruction. The dough made of sand and glue that had lent support now seemed to have a soul capable of accepting and modulating the intensity of the color, mimicking in the material the functions of the maternal psychic container. The possibility of actively correcting the result through jets of water legitimized the expression of something that seemed excessive; modulating the saturation of color thus became a gesture that could restore to her, at least partially, the legitimacy of her feelings.

We talked about the work as it gradually began to take shape and also about Violet's fear every time something inconvenient happened. Going beyond the edges of the dough or the drips of glue on the table sometimes caused Violet to freeze, manifested at times as indifference and at other times an excessive worry. When I felt able to introduce the topic of reactions to what occurred more explicitly – particularly the anger – Violet spoke for the first time of her difficult relationship with her brother (mother), who she felt did not know how to respect limits and continually invaded her space.

I thought that Violet's conflict with her brother helped her to legitimize her rage toward her mother, which felt in the past as rather inaccessible. In the present, her rage helped her understand her feeling shut out of her maternal relationship in failing to conform to their mother's expectations.

I thought that having allowed Violet to enter the adult therapy room and experience reproducing and transforming something of mine, scratching and coloring it and then erasing part of the color, must have had an impact on the psychic process of being. I thought that Violet might have experienced a new relationship with her internal mother, able to experience both the 'feminine' aspects of being one and the 'masculine' aspects of being active and different from the other. I hypothesize that the process described was in touch with the inner level of development described by Winnicott.

## Selfies: At a Crossroad with the Analyst's Culture

After about a year, as she spoke of selfies that she and her friends loved to exchange via social media, Violet suddenly and without connection to our conversation asked me a very disconcerting question: 'The pictures in the other room – are they your selfies?' Jokingly, I answered that they could be Paleozoic selfies adapted to someone of my age, given that they were painted on stone. But inside, I asked myself how she could have raised this question without knowing that I had painted the images. She laughed at my response, but evidently, she had noticed my surprise and the emotions that had flashed through me. To reinforce and not renounce her intuitive perception, she added: 'The woman inside the frame looks like you.'

The figure represented did not look like me at all, and I had never thought of doing a true self-portrait, but the starting point from which I had taken the idea for the frame/prison had been a mirror. I said nothing of this, of course, but it upset me that Violet was so closely in contact with something of mine and remembered so precisely what she had seen for only a few minutes a year earlier.

Violet proposed a return to painting in order to show me something she had learned at school during art class. She took a sheet of paper and used Scotch tape to delineate a series of stripes. Then she painted some irregular squares with a sponge, wanting to use pink and purple for her colors, and at the end, she took away the tape. 'Look,' she said to me, 'it looks a little like your frame.' I said, 'So this is sort of a selfie of yours.' This picture inaugurated a period of investigation and reflection about borders of the self and those between self and other, and how 'to be annoyed' makes relationships difficult – or sometimes it can tear them apart, as had happened with the support of the paper when the tape was torn off. 'A less adhesive Scotch is needed – paper Scotch, for example,' she suggested to me.

This expression is a nice layman's definition of what Bion calls the *invariant*: the possibility that between transformations brought about by the analyst (Ta) and those brought about by the patient (Tp), one can find an emotional continuity that guarantees the understanding and development of the psychic container (Bion, 1965, 9–144).

The use of two colors near each other from a chromatic point of view (pink and purple) and their clear distinction through white lines can be seen as an aesthetic investigation into the experience of continuity and separation. In addition, the tears in the supporting paper highlighted how Violet's rage produced analogous painful tears in the affective continuity with her mother and how these exposed her to gradually feeling fragile and incapable.

Wanting to preserve her work, Violet then passed a layer of transparent glue over the surface, which gave it brightness and textural consistency, reaffirming that greater closeness guarantees solidity. We spoke in the concrete, of course, but a reflection on how the same kinds of materials (paper on paper) could better relate to each other – just as how anger (getting annoyed) could produce holes – went beyond technical aspects. To be united, to be separated, to stick together and to be torn apart, through action, assumed a dimension of great depth. Violet found it impossible to criticize her mother during this phase of adolescence, choosing her brother as the target of her aggressiveness. Her sense of solitude and lack of value did not permit her to move about fluidly in her feminine and masculine parts. Moreover, the stigmatization of her aggressiveness as intolerable deprived her of the experience of containment in the family context. Violet felt left alone by a mother who projected into her daughter her own unthinking anxieties. Her father had difficulty taking an active role, and her brother had become the object of her aggression.

In this second clinical moment, the analysis entered a phase of development in which the patient tried to differentiate herself from the mother, experiencing the need to be connected and different at the same time. But, again, the mother projections and her personal and cultural ideas about gender disturbed the process in Violet's mind.

Exploring the border with me and the possibility of using aggression healthily gave her a chance to recreate the object in the transitional space between inside and outside. At this level, the issue of gender emerged in a complex, 'softly assembled' encounter with seeing and being seen, desire and being desired (Harris, 2016)

### Nail Polish: The Feminine at a Crossroad with the Family's Culture

A third phase of the working-through of these themes occurred through Violet's passion for nail polish and for make-up in general. Make-up was a battlefield with her mother, who countermanded her requests not only with prohibition but also with a moral judgment. Even if make-up is an appropriate way for a teenage girl to present herself, Violet's mother thought it connoted her daughter as a girl of 'easy virtue.' Violet wanted to strengthen her nails and, at the same time, beautify them, almost to the point of setting up inside herself the paradox of wanting and not wanting to use her aggression to differentiate herself from her mother. Moreover, the painted nails gave her a feeling of belonging to her group of friends.

One day, Violet arrived for her session with some bottles of nail polish that she had acquired in earlier months, but – not being able to use them or not feeling that she could legitimately use them – she found that merely looking at them aroused intense anger in her. She asked me if I would keep them until she decided to pour them down the toilet. Why empty them into such a specific container and not simply throw them away? In analysis, Violet sought a container for a part of herself that was considered unacceptable. At the same time, she did not want to be impulsive and collude with her mother's judgment that nail polish (and anger) had to be likened to excrement. She wanted our relationship to be capable of representing a temporary lapse of time that was useful for understanding.

Violet tried to paint her nails in my consulting room as though she might have a place in which to transgress mother's judgment. Her difficulty using her left hand (the smudging due to the non-dominant hand's motoric imprecision) brought her to intense anger in the session. At first, I felt this impossibility of her hands being interchangeable as a physical representation of the frustration of doing what she wanted. Later, I thought that Violet was showing me a more adolescent level of her development: her desire to belong to her peer group and to separate herself from the family could be represented by the difficulty for her hands to work together. The mother's exaggerated fear of losing her daughter's infancy and probably her difficulty with the male gender left Violet feeling guilty for the aggressive impulse useful to separate herself from her mother.

Violet felt guilt at the nail polish, according to the mother's perspective, and saw it as something good for herself to improve her feminine identity. But, moreover, the choice of the nails as the body part to express conflict let me see them as defensive and aggressive parts in a fight inside herself.

In subsequent sessions, Violet wanted to do experiments with nail polish. She let the liquid from the little bottles drip onto a sheet of paper like drops of blood, creating a mark that she then shaped with a stick as though to test its consistency. We next filled a sink with water, and Violet emptied the bottles of nail polish, creating a marbled liquid image. She told me that it looked like a screensaver on her cell phone that she liked, an image she wanted to 'capture' with the help of a sheet of paper. Her association with a screen saver implied to me a crossroad between her need to use her phone to be in contact with her friends and her existence within her family.

The marks that emerged on paper were satisfactory and surprising, and the aesthetic effect of their combination appeared to her to be an instance of 'getting on well together.' She chose to hang some pink ones and some dark blue ones from a series of these works, lining them up together in a regular way. The colors made me think again of gender and of the pink and blue bows that are hung on the outside of a front door when there has been a birth. Violet's works appeared to me to represent the birth of a possible balance of the masculine and the feminine within her and a newly born desire to be able to show this accomplishment to the outside world.

### 'Transitory Objects'

The unique feature of the therapeutic journey with Violet was that we were able to meet in an intersubjective field where something common to our subjectivation as females could be recognized and become useful in the therapy. The beginning of a meaningful emotional transformation started through images present in my consulting room and then through other ones produced in the treatment.

Images root in sensations more than words can. Images are the ground floor of identity and representation; for this reason, I chose to describe the previous images as pivotal in redefining Violet's feminine identity as the treatment progressed. The use of painting was not primarily a way to explore feeling, as in art therapy. Rather, from a Field Theory perspective, the use of the images let Violet and me enter into a particular field of sharing.

The pictures described in the first phase of therapy allowed a state of sharing in which there was no distance, no clarity between here and there. Through Violet's first images about the body (evoked by my paintings), we started to explore something of primary femininity. An area in which something happened in the tie that ensures going on being, a place where a primary link has been broken, perhaps in the mother, certainly between the mother and child.

These paintings produced by the patient and with the elaborations described previously in the second and third phases of therapy allowed us to explore the adolescent process. This redefinition expanded Violet's experience of gender identity, including influences derived from her familial and societal gender culture.

In contrast to the *transitional objects* described by Winnicott (which represent a meeting between self and not-self and which define an area of play and illusion), *transitory objects* have the function of sketching out a sort of map between disorganizing areas of self and their relational side. An area that Winnicott described as early, unconscious ruptures – 'breaks in unity' different than the usual process of differentiation in development. Because these experiences are out of meaning, they are a developmental unfolding of experience (sensations outside of conscious memory) and an unfolding of representation. Botella and Botella's theory (2015) about figurability offers a fit description of the emergence of these types of experiences during therapy. Bion (1962) named this type of experience "waking dream thoughts," by which he intended to describe a continuous transformation of raw sensations and proto-emotions into narrative derivates. We can imagine gender and desire as aspects of experiences of 'going on' becoming 'figurable' or real daydreams that can become unconscious (Civitarese, 2011).

Objects with high sensory potential (such as plastic and color) are able to recreate a bodily and emotional transit rich in sign and movement. The creation of transitory objects permitted the integration of masculine (going on) and feminine (being) parts of the patient and a transformation of the therapeutic relationship as the external side of this integration.

## Discussion

The pathological connotation that Violet's mother attributed to her daughter's push to become a subject left Violet feeling marginalized in their relationship. This added a sense of growing frustration, of rejection of her own knowledge, to her original aggression. The social and cultural container, in addition to the maternal one, brought home to Violet that being aggressive was not appropriate for being female. This experience pushed her toward submissive behavior in social relationships. In addition to personal aspects, subsequent events (cultural or performative, as Butler defines them)[5] widened the gap between the masculine modality and the feminine one of being in relation to the other.

The hypothesis of this contribution is that when a cultural attitude that tends to pathologize the expression of feminine aggression is emphasized within the family, a specific alteration in psychic development results. Using Bion's symbolism, one can hypothesize that the missed experience of being contained in the mind of the other might produce a deformation in the development of the psychic container. Stigmatization of normal aggression as a pathological element produces in the adolescent an alteration in this psychic function, which manifests as confusion, an inability to decide or a violent expulsion of rage through acting out. Through the previously mentioned material, we intended to show this psychic difficulty.

We also intended to show how some aesthetic tools, which we term '*transitory objects,*' can be used, particularly in adolescence, to restore psychic functioning. Feeling marginalized has a double edge: the margins are where feelings of uncertainty or insecurity tend to flourish but may allow a creative point of view. Mother's projection into her daughter caused Violet to feel wrong for her mother – angry, un-contained and on the margins. The key question isn't how to eliminate this feeling but how to ride it. Transitory objects aren't necessarily art objects but relational tools able to promote the transition from the sorrow of relational disconnection to connectedness.

From a Field Theory perspective, the analyst has to put aside the real relational story of the patient to focus on what happens between analyst and patient (Ferro & Civitarese, 2015; Molinari, 2017). The flow of the transitory objects improves the capacity to transform sensations and raw emotions into a waking dreaming. From this point of view, Violet's artworks were not any artistic expression but were triggered by her analyst's paintings created during her own analysis, a very personal expression captured by Violet with great sensibility. The patient's use of the 'objects' posed by the analyst and the analyst's openness to offer part of her experience in a symbolic form (to use the analyst herself as an object in Winnicott's sense) are moments of extreme fertility that reinforce our confidence in a non-omnipotent, sensitive psychoanalysis.

The old question of how the gender of the analyst helps or hinders the process is always present. This is not a simple question to answer because it is not obvious that analyst and patient being of the same sex would facilitate the process. The fertility of the couple depends on many factors other than gender: the space offered and co-created, where feelings can be contained and find limits that allow them to be transformed in a non-accusatory climate. But can we deny that femininity has its particularities that only two women can share? And that two men also share particularities?

Abandoning an old psychoanalytic view that might consider separation a goal of subject development and observing the process that transitory objects allow, we can learn something more. We can observe how unconscious connections between minds – between individuals – determine what we know, how we know and the vastly complex fields within which we affect each other in analysis and in culture. The images found in the analyst's studio and those produced by Violet represented, to a certain extent, a 'subjective object' for each and, at the same time, the *thinking surface* of their meetings.

Violet's hatred toward her twin brother must not be understood as a simple relational difficulty but as rage at not feeling herself centered enough in the maternal mind. The maternal fear of that rage marginalized Violet compared to her brother, generating further demanding and violent behaviors, difficult to decode or accept.

It can be posited that from the beginning, twins have different intrauterine experiences. Their preferred positions and interactions may also affect their relationship after birth (Piontelli, 1989, 417). After birth, mother could give attention unconsciously more to one twin than the other. This can be due to a weaker baby or one that is more active (Piontelli, 2002). Each twin may be very jealous of the attention the other receives from their mother. Sometimes, the access to maternal care is more difficult for twins, which strengthens the relationship between them so that, over time, they tend to consolidate complementary modes that produce a strong relationship. In other situations, particularly if mother struggles to maintain a balanced triangular relationship, the twins take on roles designed to meet maternal expectations and remain in competition with each other in a harsh way (Stewart, 2003).

Violet seemed to have taken on the mother's narcissistic sufferings and the angry disappointment toward the male twin. This did not allow her to internalize the male part, active and distant, integrating it with her own delicate, sensitive parts. She described her brother as intrusive and unable to respect limits. Violet's difficulty seemed to be rooted in an early stage of development of gender identity and relationship with the other. However, she was also on the threshold of adolescence, a time of life when the reshaping of the relationship with the parents and peers, as well as the influence of culture, had an important influence on the building of gender identity.

The therapeutic restitution of an experience of recognition, then, had to traverse two realms: the emotional one of anger and that of a relational practice aimed at modifying the *performative* or cultural aspects that influence gender identity, of which the parents are the natural means of transmission. Confusion and submission, in the final analysis, are the desires of the oppressed, and in this mother-daughter relationship, they are the epiphenomenon of the frustration of an intimate closeness. The non-acceptance of anger at a certain stage is shown to amputate the development of the container function, increasing projection as a defense.

Inclusion in the analytic relationship of an artistic experience and the creation of *transitory objects* may sustain the integration of body and mind in the specifics of the therapeutic relationship with an adolescent.

As many artists testify, during the development of an artwork, the piece acquires a 'presence' that can affect the direction of the work. In the described case, the transformation into paintings represents something about the transformation process of analyst and patient while living and thinking together conscious and unconscious parts of their experience, as a living daydreaming. In so doing, the creative process needs integration of destructiveness, aggression and the ability to build new forms (Townsend, 2015). Moreover, the internal creative process had to face the aggression that an imaginary audience may not approve of the new creation. (Parker, 1998). So, the transitory object may be the space of playing and mending, allowing the emotional experience to cross different levels of experience: the body-based inter-affectivity (Boston Change Process Study Group <BCPSG>, 2018), the unconscious intersubjective space, the creative construction of new meanings.

The aesthetic aspects belonging to the birth of the body-mind then functioned as vectors for the birth of little 'affective padlocks,' an expression of the social body-mind.[6]

## Final Considerations

Freud warned: "[I]t is important to understand that the concepts of feminine and masculine, whose meanings seem so free from ambiguities for ordinary people, are among the most confused in science" (1905, 226). Now, we know that the developmental processes intersect and interact with the subject's experiences of sexuality and desire, parents' wishes and culture; all these issues determine complex and changing gender identifications (Caldwell, 2007; Chodorow, 1989; Butler, 1990; Benjamin, 1998; Dimen, 2003; Dimen & Goldner, 2007; Corbett, 2011; Corbett et al., 2014; Harris, 1997, 2002)

The clinical work presented here approaches the feminine/masculine subject starting from Winnicott's concepts of the creative constitution of the psyche. Winnicott contemplates the necessity of 'being' (feminine) and 'doing' (masculine) as essential elements for mental development. At the beginning of Winnicott's work, feminine and masculine are not directly related to gender; he used them in the same way Bion used feminine and masculine to refer to the container and contained. Later, in his work "On the split-off male and female elements" (1971), he addressed the complexity of bi-gender in psychic life and opened a new way of thinking about the process by which gender may emerge. In establishing first being and doing, sexuality becomes entangled with the parent's desire imbued with their conscious and unconscious subjective expectations. The possibility for traumatic effects is in the explicit messages sent to the child from the parents' projections and projective identifications. Enigmatic messages condition sexuality and identity during the developmental process. When these messages are massive and interfere with other features, such as biological predisposition, the quality of attachment, the presence of significant figures beyond parents and gender trauma (Saketopoulou, 2014) can result.

The clinical case presented in this paper doesn't show massive gender trauma. Rather, it allows us to see how the earliest mother and child links are an essential conduit for intergenerational transmissions about gender identity as well as the impact during adolescence when the role of society becomes more relevant.

Adolescence becomes a crucial time in development when the unconscious aspects of the parental message have a chance of transformation. But, of course, elements of these ongoing message transmissions were beyond Violet's mentalizing capacities. Still, cognitive development, active sexual desire and the crucial task of differentiation make adolescence a time of possible retranslation of these messages.

Psychoanalysis explores issues of gender and sexuality and how they shape the evolution of intersubjectivity. The immediacy of the immersive perceptive moment can allow embodied feeling states to emerge, where the gap between these forms and their context becomes crucial for new meaning. Contemporary psychoanalysis is as receptive to absence as presence and explores how presence is always an interplay between what becomes and what is not yet present.

We tried to focus on the transformative point in which the intersection of the patient's and the analyst's experiences found boundaries and started going toward differentiation.

Both the analyst and the patient had to do unconscious work to transform the understandable need for recognition, which had been damaged by maternal projections.

## Notes

1 Representability is also the work of adults in analysis, for instance, in integrating new experiences of pregnancy, aging or illness. Such new experiences require emotional work to make meaning of them.
2 There are similarities between the Barangers and Italian Field Theorists such as Ferro, Civitarese and Molinari. For instance, Italian Field Theorists particularly emphasize Bion's development of the importance of unsaturated interpretations and the continued creation of new meanings.
3 The analyst of this case is Elena Molinari.
4 Jannis Kounellis is a contemporary artist who was born in Greece and then moved to Italy, where he became part of the Arte Povera school.
5 Butler defines *performative* as a repetitive act, anchored in culture, that renders gender norms unavoidable and ongoing. In this sense, culture would function with the same structural mandate as language (Butler, 1990).
6 We refer here to the thousands of teenagers who copy the protagonists of Federico Moccia's (2006) bestseller *I Want You* by attaching padlocks to bridges as a sign of eternal love.

## References

Anagnostaki, L., Zaharia, A., & Matsouka, M. (2017). Discussing the therapeutic setting in child and adolescent psychoanalytic psychotherapy. *Journal of Child Psychotherapy*, 43(3), 369–379.

Baranger, M., & Baranger, W. (2008). The analytic situation as a dynamic field, trans. S. Rogers & J. Churcher. *The International Journal of Psychoanalysis*, 89(4), 795–826. (Original work published 1961.)

Benjamin, J. (1998). *The Bonds of Love: Psychoanalysis, Feminism, and the Problem of Domination*. New York: Pantheon.

Bion, W.R. (1961). *Experiences in Groups.* London: Tavistock.

Bion, W.R. (1962). *Learning from Experience.* London: William Heinemann.

Bion, W.R. (1965). *Transformations.* London: William Heinemann.

Bion, W.R. (1970). *Attention and Interpretation.* London: Tavistock.

Bion, W.R. (2013). Notes on memory and desire. In J. Aguayo & B. Malin (Eds.), *Wilfred Bion: Los Angeles Seminars and Supervision* (pp. 136–138). London: Karnac. (Original work published 1967.)

Boston Change Process Study Group. (2018). Moving through and being moved by: Embodiment in development and in the therapeutic relationship. *Contemporary Psychoanalysis,* 54, 299–321.

Brady, M.T. (2018). *Analytic Engagements with Adolescents: Sex, Gender and Subversion.* Abingdon & New York, NY: Routledge.

Butler, J. (1990). *Gender Trouble: Feminism and the Subversive Identity.* New York, NY: Routledge.

Caldwell, L. (2007). Being and sexuality: Contribution or confusion? In L. Caldwell (Ed.), *Winnicott and the Psychoanalytic Tradition.* London: Karnac.

Chodorow, N. (1989). *Feminism and Psychoanalytic Theory.* New Haven, CT: Yale University Press.

Civitarese, G. (2011). Exploring core concepts: Sexuality, dreams and the unconscious. *International Journal of Psychoanalysis,* 92, 277–280.

Corbett, K. (2011). Gender regulation. *Psychoanalytic Quarterly,* 80, 441–459.

Corbett, K., Dimen, M., Goldner, V., & Harris, A. (2014). Talking sex, talking gender – A roundtable. *Studies in Gender and Sexuality,* 15, 295–317.

Dimen, M. (2003). *Sexuality, Intimacy, Power.* Hillsdale, NJ: The Analytic Press.

Dimen, M., & Goldner, V. (2007). *Gender in Psychoanalytic Space.* New York: Other Press.

Ferro, A. (2018). Bionian and post-bionian transformations. *Revue Roumaine de Psychanalyse,* 11, 47–56.

Ferro, A., & Civitarese, G. (2015). *The Analytic Field and Its Transformations.* London: Karnac.

Freud, S. (1905). Three essays on the theory of sexuality. *SE,* VII, 123–243.

Grotstein, J. (2011). *The Psychoanalytic Covenant: The Hidden Order of Transference and Countertransference.* 2011 Franz Alexander Lecture, Sponsored by the New Center for Psychoanalysis, Friday, March 25, 2011.

Harris, A. (1997). Aggression, envy, and ambition: Circulating tensions in women's psychic life. *Gender and Psychoanalysis,* 2, 291–325.

Harris, A. (2002). Mothers, monsters, mentors. *Studies in Gender and Sexuality,* 3, 281–295.

Harris, A. (2016). Winnicott and gender madness. *British Journal of Psychotherapy,* 32(3), 359–375.

Laor, I.M.A. (2007). The therapist, the patient, and the therapeutic setting: Mutual construction of the setting as a therapeutic factor. *Psychoanalytic Dialogues,* 17(1), 29–46.

Moccia, F. (2006). *Ho voglia di te (I Want You).* Milano: Feltrinelli.

Molinari, E. (2017). *Field Theory in Child and Adolescent Psychoanalysis: Understanding and Reacting to Unexpected Developments.* Abingdon & New York, NY: Routledge.

Obholzer, A. (1996). Psychoanalytic contributions to authority and leadership issues. *The Leadership & Organization Development Journal,* 17(6).

Parker, R. (1998). Killing the angel in the house: Creativity, femininity and aggression. *International Journal of Psychoanalysis,* 79, 757–774.

Piontelli, A. (1989). A study on twins before or after birth. *International Review of Psych-Analysis,* 16, 413–426.

Piontelli, A. (2002). *Twins: From Foetus to Child.* London & New York, NY: Routledge.

Saketopoulou, A. (2014). Mourning the body as bedrock: Development considerations in treating transsexual patients analytically. *Journal of the American Psychoanalytic Association,* 62, 773–806.

Stefana, A., & Gamba, A. (2018). From the "squiggle game" to "games of reciprocity" towards a creative co-construction of a space for working with adolescents. *The International Journal of Psychoanalysis*, 99(2), 355–379.

Stewart, H (2003). Winnicott, Balint, and the independent tradition. *The American Journal of Psychoanalysis*, 63(3), 207–217.

Townsend, P. (2015). Creativity and destructiveness in art and psychoanalysis. *British Journal of Psychotherapy*, 31(1), 120–131.

Winnicott, D. (1971). On the split-off male and female elements. In *Playing and Reality*. London: Tavistock.

Winnicott, D. (1989) The fate of the transitional object. In C. Winnicott, R. Shepherd, & M. Davis (Eds.), *Psycho-Analytic Explorations* (pp. 53–58). Karnac Books Ltd. (Original work published 1959.)

Winnicott, D. (1989). On the split-off male and female elements. In C. Winnicott, R. Shepherd, & M. Davis (Eds.), *Psycho-Analytic Explorations* (pp. 168–189). Karnac Books Ltd. (Original work published 1966.)

# Chapter 5

# Fear of Eating Up the Mother

## An Adolescent Phantasy in Some Anorectics

## Introduction

Eating disordered patients can be among the most difficult to treat. They present analysts with potentially life-threatening crises and the possible need for substantial ancillary care. Even more challenging is their form of primitive bodily communication. This bodily communication needs to emerge in the analytic relationship – such as in binge-like modes of relating (which bypass the possibility of real nourishment) or anorexic indifference to the analyst and the sessions. The emergence of these symptomatic communications in the analysis is fraught but provides an opportunity for the unconscious bodily and relational phantasies underlying the symptoms to begin to be known.

The body expresses what the mind cannot contain at all ages, but particularly in adolescence (Brady, 2016). The pressures of puberty and rapid bodily change can overwhelm the mind's capacity to assimilate them. Eating disorders are part of the broad range of psychosomatic disorders that tend to emerge in adolescence and often persist long after. This chapter discusses (in the metaphor of this book) a breakdown in 'surfing' in the rigidified restrictions of the anorexic adolescent, trapped instead in a fortress body with the drawbridge drawn up.

Many issues need to be considered in relation to the development of an eating disorder: as representing problems with identity and the construction of a self (Brady, 2011); as a rejection of pubertal development (Anderson, 2005); as a disturbed effort to separate and individuate from mother and paradoxically also to prevent separation from mother (Rey, 1994); as a bodily expression of unbearable psychic pain (Burloux, 2005); as an effort to keep out intolerable parental projections (Williams, 1997); as an expression of self-destruction and as an urgent communication. In many patients, some or all of these dynamics are intertwined.

Bion (1962) emphasizes that digestion is not a metaphor, but rather that the mind develops around experiences of digestion, which are so fundamental to life. Child analysts are very familiar with disturbances in eating and the associated unconscious phantasies related to eating in children. A child's horror at different foods on her plate touching, at the mushiness of boiled carrots, the 'skin' on top of the pudding or at eating meat may seem amusing to adults, but indicates the deep

DOI: 10.4324/9781003498810-6

meanings in eating. Biting and chewing can be experienced as pleasurable but also as destructive. The eating symptoms in eating disorders can be dramatic, but they can be extreme forms of anxiety in us all. Eating disorders must also be understood as part of far more pervasive problems in taking in and relating.

In this chapter, I will focus on the unconscious phantasy that eating and growing destroys the mother, which Henri Rey (1994) has detailed. Rey was a psychoanalyst in London who spent much of his professional life at the Maudsley Hospital, treating borderline and psychotic patients. He had a great deal of experience in the treatment of anorexia nervosa.

I will first describe Rey's supervision of the treatment of a 19-year-old hospitalized anorexic female, 'Miss R.' Rey's groundbreaking writing on anorexia depicted the treatment of female patients, although he was well aware of anorexia in males (1994). I have chosen to discuss Rey's work because it is not widely known among clinicians of adolescents. Steiner comments that:

> Despite his French ebullience Henri Rey was a shy man and he did not give a paper in the psychoanalytic society until he had retired. He was nevertheless greatly influenced by his analysis with Herbert Rosenfeld and his supervision with Joan Riviere. His ideas are not as well-known as they should be and his major work, *Universals of Psychoanalysis in the Treatment of Psychotic and Borderline States*, was not published until 1994 and has yet to be fully assimilated by psychiatrists and psychoanalysts.
>
> (Steiner, 2012)

In addition to his insight into psychotic and borderline states, I have been struck by Rey's profound understanding of adolescent separation processes, which is conveyed in his work on anorexia. Steiner rightly notes that Rey "always remembered the importance of the body and of the body schema in the mental organization" (p. xi, Foreword in Rey, 1994).

## Rey's Conceptualization of Anorexia Nervosa

### Rey's Miss R.[1]

'Miss R.' was a severely anorexic 19-year-old, weighing only 72 lbs. when she was admitted to the hospital. She was near death and required intravenous hydration and tube feeding. One striking element was that she was happy to receive feeding through the tube but had an intense aversion to chewing or swallowing food. This finding makes me wonder if Miss R. was not opposed to living, or even to being closer to normal weight, but was horrified at having any active responsibility for eating, including chewing and swallowing.

Rey described Miss R. as a highly intelligent college student majoring in psychology. She wrote up her own experiences of treatment (Rouah, 1980). Rey saw the process of writing as contributing to her development of symbolic function and away from the concrete expression of her eating disorder. Through his understanding of Miss R., Rey details what he views as the central problem in anorexia nervosa – becoming an adult implies eating the mother to grow up. In anorexia, food is experienced very concretely by the mother.

The onset of Miss R.'s illness was at puberty. She related, "[T]he changes of pubescence, the increase in size, shape and weight, menstruation and new and disturbing sexual impulses, all presented a dangerous challenge for which I was unprepared and which thwarted what little control I had" (quoted by Rey, p. 48). Rey theorized that "at puberty Miss R started controlling food to prevent heterosexual impulses, to prevent womanhood, and to reduce her body to childlike proportions. That is, she tried to prevent all desires and possibilities of becoming pregnant" (p. 63).

Miss R.'s mother had been orphaned at an early age and was described as childlike. Father had been a dominant personality, but shortly before entering puberty, Miss R. witnessed his sudden death by cardiac arrest. Mother insisted on enshrining father's clothing and other items exactly as they had been before father died, leaving Miss. R. to feel she was alone in coping with father's death. Her loss of her father and her mother's absorption in her grief left Miss R. psychically isolated (Brady, 2015a) and thrown back on her body to the only place to express her troubles.

### Phantasies About Eating

While hospitalized, Miss R. made a series of remarkable drawings conveying her sense of eating as violent and destructive of her object. One is entitled 'The Chick and the Shell' about which she says, "the baby is like a little chick who grows by eating all the reserves in the egg until there is nothing left except the empty dried-out useless shell which it will shatter open, and step out of as a fully grown individual, ungratefully leaving the shell behind, this shell which once fed and protected it." She conveys her sense of eating and the growth it causes as hostile. We could also surmise that she experienced her mother as debilitated and weak, and so there would be no lively mother to stand in useful contrast to these phantasies. Clearly, she experiences eating and growing as a 'zero sum game,' in which one gains and one loses. She seems to have no sense that a mother could feel enhanced or enriched by her adolescent daughter's growth while also feeling some loss.

Miss R. entitles another series of drawings, "The Parasite and Tree." The drawings depict a large tree shedding its seeds, a small tree growing and the original tree withering and dying. Miss R. relates: "[T]he parasite has grown and flourished at the host's expense. It has selfishly sucked up all the goodness out of the tree whose resources are now completely exhausted" (p. 51). These drawings powerfully convey Miss. R.'s harsh superego and her phantasy of destroying her mother through greed and by growing up.

In a post-Bionian framework, Miss R. is developing narratives through her drawings and stories which contribute to the growth of a mind that can begin to contain and metabolize previously uncontained, concrete elements. Ferro (1999) would describe this as developing 'narrative derivatives' that enhance the ability of the mind to make meaning. What was previously left to the body to speak could now begin to take symbolic form in Miss R.'s mind. Her thoughts and feelings could begin to be understood by others, thus lessening the isolative hold of anorexia. We see the development of a narrative with a therapeutic other, beginning to allow other methods of communication than the bodily and for the development of object relations outside the 'zero sum game.'

Miss R. details a link in her mind between her fear of obesity and her childhood phantasy that pregnant women swallow their babies. She conveys her view that 'obesity' can be for one of two reasons, overeating or pregnancy:

([]n the first case, eating and indulging in food would result in a fat, and to my mind, an ugly and repulsive figure. In the second instance, my phantasy involves that of a foetus being cut up and chewed like food, swallowed hence landing up in mother's stomach where it would grow and result in the mother's obese appearance. This, the common denominator of the two subparts of my phantasy, is the resulting state of the individual (obesity) which scares me. This had led me to hypothesize the possibility that subconsciously I equate food with a baby being swallowed which to my mind is a barbaric and repulsive act.

(53)

In order to comprehend Miss R.'s phantasies it is important to remember that the fundamental principle of functioning in the paranoid-schizoid position is the law of the talion, that is, 'an eye for an eye' or here, eat and you will be eaten. In a schizoid mentality (Segal, 1964), the punishment fits the crime in a very concrete manner. The possibilities of the depressive position, such as forgiveness, compassion or true reparation, are not available.

Rey contends that by the projection of her own greed, the anorexic believes that the baby has gotten inside the mother because the mother has devoured the baby. He felt it essential to "insist on the anorectic's wish to do the right thing, that thinking as she does is right, granted she thinks as she does . . . (p. 66). Rey suggests that in anorexia, the inability to symbolize can be specific to the system of food and body (size) in patients who are quite able to symbolize in other areas. Another way of putting this is that thinking capacities can be overwhelmed by fraught emotions involving the body and separation processes. Rey saw the development of anorexia as beginning to be able to conceive of other meanings to eating than that of eating mother or of oneself being eaten.

As 'Natalia,' a 22-year-old patient of mine, prepared to leave treatment to move away for graduate school, she spoke of being terrified about the idea of having a baby. Her associations had a science fiction film quality, replete with parasitic images of breastfeeding. I thought that she felt quite frightened of knowing about all her feelings of need for me as she left. She was leaving treatment before she was really ready to end. I thought her need to get out from under mother figures was partly motivated by her desire for us. This sort of departure is common in late adolescents/young adults, where it is so developmentally appropriate to separate from parental figures, make changes, and reach for new abilities. There was much in her departure that felt developmentally progressive. At the same time, I thought Natalia was telling me that she felt afraid of a damaging baby self that needed more help. (This case is discussed at greater length in Brady, 2015b).

Rey says:

> This creation of the baby-eating mother is clearly a projective identification of the baby into the mother. The problem for the anorectic is how to be a growing foetus without eating the mother . . . and, in the identification with the mother, not to eat the baby to become pregnant.
>
> (p. 64)

Rey saw anorexics as tortured by the dilemma of needing to eat and yet believing eating to be destructive. The interpretation of this dilemma allows an anorectic patient to begin to consider the functioning of his/her own mind rather than only being locked into the control of the body.

Rey's observation that the anorexic patient needs "an actual 'acting out' as near as possible to reality to work through her fundamental conflict" (p. 64) seems to me particularly cogent. The anorexic brings her problems to us in a very concrete manner and her communication needs to be accepted at this level until other modes of communication become possible. In fact, anorexics have often so withdrawn into bodily communication that their capacity to conceive of or relate emotions is stunted. The analytic expectation of interactions that convey emotional meaning is something some anorexics don't understand.

### Bodily Phantasies

In accordance with her eating phantasies, Rey relates that Miss R. was preoccupied with her body image, desiring the body of a child or even a fetus. Distortion of body image is a common denominator of anorexia. Anorexics insist that they are overweight when, to others' eyes, they look emaciated. Being underweight is necessary to fend off the self-accusations of having greedily eaten up the mother. Rey's insight that anorexia can be a defense against bulimia is clinically very useful, understanding that the patient is trying to save both her mother and herself from being devoured. From another vantage point, Miss R. also felt that her body had a false, misleading outer shell – she wanted to cut out eating to expose her child self. Here, the child self is equated with innocence, but Miss R. also needed her child self to be seen in order to help her have a way forward that wasn't false.

The distorting effect on body image through the equation of smallness with innocence reaches delusional proportions in anorexics. Rey sees the development out of anorexia as involving the treatment of these delusions – first in regard to the formation of symbols and their use, second in interpretation in the transference.

Rey observed that the anorectics he worked with:

> . . . always began to get better when they started using 'symbols' of one kind or another. I realized that they could not come out of their 'delusional system'

without a metasystem into which to project and integrate and transform the material into a higher system than the delusional one.

(p. 67).

Some anorexic patients are quite capable of complex symbolic thought, but not in relation to food and size. Rey saw Miss R.'s projective art and writing while hospitalized as promoting her capacity for symbolization, and one could also say for creativity.

This is similar to child analysis, in which the play in play therapy can allow the elaboration of narrative derivatives and the growth of the mind, which I will discuss in the next chapter. "[O]nce the transference has started, the delusional phantasies and beliefs can be compared to the interpretations of the therapist" (p. 68). In the meantime, keeping the patient alive is important. Rey considers that it is through transference love, in part evoked by the effort to keep the patient alive and through the acceptance of her infantile needs, "that the fortress inside the patient begins to yield" (p. 68). From fortress towards 'learning to surf.'

## Note

1 The material in this section is from Rey, 1994.

## References

Anderson, R. (2005). Adolescence and the body ego: The reencountering of primitive mental functioning in adolescent development. Unpublished paper presented at *The Sixteenth Annual Melanie Klein Memorial Lectureship*, January 8, 2005, Los Angeles.

Bion, W.R. (1962). *Learning from Experience*. London: Heinemann.

Brady, M.T. (2011). Invisibility and insubstantiality in an anorexic adolescent: Phenomenology and dynamics. *Journal of Child Psychotherapy*, 37(1), 3–15.

Brady, M.T. (2015a). 'Unjoined persons': Psychic isolation in adolescence and its relation to bodily symptoms. *Journal of Child Psychotherapy*, 41, 179–194.

Brady, M.T. (2015b). High up on bar stools: Manic defences and an oblivious object in a late adolescent. *Journal of Child Psychotherapy*, 41(1), 52–72.

Brady, M.T. (2016). *The Body in Adolescence: Psychic Isolation and Physical Symptoms*. New York, NY: Routledge.

Burloux, G. (2005). *The Body and Its Pain*. Free Association Books.

Ferro, A. (1999). *The Bi-Personal Field: Experiences in Child Analysis*. London & New York, NY: Routledge.

Rey, H. (1994). Anorexia nervosa. In *Universals of Psychoanalysis in the Treatment of Psychotic and Borderline States*. London: Free Association Books.

Rouah, A. (1980). Anorexia nervosa. *Psychotherapia*, 6, 17–25.

Segal, H. (1964). *An Introduction to the Work of Melanie Klein*. New York: Basic Books, Inc., Publishers.

Steiner, J. (2012). *Henri Rey*. Melanie Klein Trust. www.melanie-klein-trust.org.uk/rey

Williams, G. (1997). Reflections on some dynamics of eating disorders: 'No entry' defenses and foreign bodies. *International Journal of Psycho-Analysis*, 78, 927–941.

Chapter 6

# To Know or Not to Know

## An Application of Bion's K and −K to Child Treatment

*Mary T. Brady, Robert Tyminski and Kristen Carey*

### Introduction

Bion did not treat children, yet many of his interrelated concepts, such as container/ contained, maternal reverie, and the development of thinking through alpha function, are highly applicable to child treatment. Additionally, his conceptualizations of thinking and non-thinking states (K or −K links) underlie the possibility for development in children, which is "learning from experience." Bion's premise that the purpose of analysis is the growth of the mind is synonymous with the child analyst's goals of fostering development and understanding impediments to development. This chapter will consider these concepts in relation to child treatment and then explicate them through the descriptions of the psychotherapies of two children: one, a vignette from a brilliant 7-year-old girl whose emotional understanding lagged far behind her intellectual capacities, and the other two sessions from a 9-year-old girl with cerebral palsy who was conceived through in vitro fertilization. Initially part of a triplet in utero, she became a twin when one fetus was spontaneously aborted. We will consider these girls' efforts to know (K) and not to know (−K) in the face of their emotional environments, complex origins, or developmental challenges.

Bion views child analysis as "extremely creative" in releasing capacities because the defenses of children are less fossilized than those of adults (2005, 55).[1] In *The Tavistock Seminars*, Bion comments that:

> people say, "It's no good to psychoanalyse a child of two or three or five." I have even heard fantastic statements about not being able to do anything when "the fibres are not myelinated." The trouble with the myelinated fibres is that the person who has them is often so rigid, so structured, that you can't get another idea through their myelin.
>
> (2005, 15)

Bion describes real contact between any two people as like a storm – capturing how unsettling it is to sense that the other person in the consulting room is completely different from oneself. For adults treating children, an added level of the foreign intensifies the storm. Ogden says that in order to read early Bion, "the reader must

DOI: 10.4324/9781003498810-7

be able to tolerate not knowing, getting lost, being confused and pressing ahead anyway" (2004a, 286). This uncertain state of mind is analogous to what a child therapist needs to sustain. Even more than with adult patients, we can lose our bearings. There is less secondary process thought. There is less of a veneer of shared social conventions. There is more action and, often, more commotion: the girl won't come into the building for her session; the boy is throwing paper airplanes at his therapist's head; the teenager's parents call to say she organized a party where Ecstasy was taken; a boy brings his boa constrictor unannounced to meet his therapist.

Bion (1970) emphasizes the differences between thinking about an experience and being in an experience. Psychoanalytic treatment of children immerses us in a dream scene brought to life in play, art, imaginary roles, action, and words. With a profound respect for the difficulty of thinking under pressure and an appreciation for our need for containment in order to be able to think, Bion says that we need to be able to "interpret under fire." The analyst of a child or adolescent is under fire much of the time. We must participate in play and react to behavior, absorbing the feelings and roles conveyed in the analytic field. At times, we might even need to physically restrain a child while struggling to retain our capacity to think.

Bion was heavily influenced by his experiences in World War I, which he entered at age 19. The devastation of combat affected him for a lifetime. Additionally, his first wife died in childbirth. After he married his second wife, Francesca, Bion had a remarkably fertile period of writing, during which he developed many of his seminal ideas, such as container/contained, a theory of thinking, and attacks on linking. This foment of theoretical development seems related in part to the safety his relationship with his wife accorded him, allowing his return to the horror of his war experience (Brown, 2012). In his own life, his personal experience of trauma, the painful difficulty of growth, and the containment that made it possible to capture the essence of Bion's thinking.

We will briefly consider Bion's interrelated concepts of maternal reverie and container/contained in relation to the development of thinking. We will then focus on the K link as a key to understanding the clinical material presented. Bion's relationship to theory is unique in that while he acknowledges its importance in allowing us to see something in a new way, he also says that we must be ready to discard theory as it can offer a false sense of understanding:

> As we try to express or formulate our findings . . . so we also excrete a kind of shell around them, a layer of knowledge that we can neither penetrate nor break out of.
>
> (Bion, 2005, 33)

## The Development of Thinking

Bion sees the first form of thinking as striving to know another emotionally. Early emotional events between a mother[2] and her infant are decisive for the capacity to think in the infant and for the possibility of growth in the mother. Bion sees thinking as a human link, as the emotional experience of trying to know oneself or another.

As is well known, Bion expanded Klein's concept of projective identification beyond its defensive uses. Klein saw projective identification as a necessary developmental step in early childhood, along with splitting, to separate dangerous, hostile impulses from loving ones (Klein, 1975/1946). That is, the badness or anxiety too difficult to experience inside the self is evacuated out into the other – sometimes by a child in the form of hyperactivity or aggression. Bion acknowledged Klein for her insights into projective identification but also took the concept in an expansive, new direction. He saw projective identification as not just a mechanism of defense but as the first mode of communication between mother and infant – as the first rudiment of thinking. The infant conveys his fears to his mother by projecting them into her for her to receive and know. The mother receives the fears and thinks about them, struggling to contain them by giving them meaning. The mother then conveys the results of her struggles and thinking by projecting them back into the infant, who introjects her metabolized thinking. Thus, the child's ability to gradually know him or herself is facilitated by being taken in and known in his mother's mind. As child therapists, we are also concerned about the support and containment that parents have or lack, as well as their internal capacities for containment. Parents are pressed hard to absorb the extreme feelings of infants and children, never mind adolescents.

## Maternal Reverie

According to Bion, maternal reverie is the capacity of the primary object to love and think about his or her infant, allowing the infant to gradually internalize a parent who is able to think and, optimally, to absorb the experience that his or her feelings can be modified, understood, and related to. Patients who have experienced little maternal reverie convey (in words or actions) that they experience their feelings as uncontestable "facts." In treatment, the therapist receives these raw, unmodulated feelings through projective identification. Bion (1962, 36) writes,

> If the feeding mother cannot allow reverie or if the reverie is allowed but is not associated with love for the child or its father this fact will be communicated to the infant even though incomprehensible to the infant.

This lack of the experience of reverie leaves the infant without the sense that experiences can be thought about or that pain and frustration can be ameliorated by love.

The analyst's reverie is, ideally, grounded in a state of mind as open as possible to experiencing what is most true for the patient and then finding words to convey something of that truth back to the patient. Some form of transformation in playing, dreaming, or thinking is only possible when the analyst takes the patient's experience in depth. Bion saw this as an endlessly courageous and creative state – the willingness to know another person, at which we are always partially failing – but pressing ahead anyway.

## Container/Contained

Bion sees the personality as constituted by two elements – contained and container – in a dynamic intercourse or relationship, with the contained continually seeking a container. Symington and Symington (1996) say, "The archetype for container/contained is mother's breast/infant" (p. 52). In an attuned relationship between a mother and baby, a sense of a loving relationship can be internalized into the infant's personality, which transforms into an internal healthy container and contained dynamic in the infant. Alternatively, in a misattuned relationship between a mother and baby, a destructive container can be internalized – for example, a punitive super-ego style containment that squashes any potential for experimental parts of the personality. Problems also result when the container is too rigid for what needs to be contained, or the contained is so explosive that the container is overwhelmed (Ferro, 1999).

Likewise, in analysis, the task of the analyst is to communicate to the patient the possibility of something new – an interaction between two people that can contain pain and result in mental growth. As the analysis progresses, optimally, this dynamic will constantly evolve. The analyst, like the mother, needs to intuit her patient's feelings by "introjecting them, sustaining them, delaying action upon them so as to modify and modulate their impact . . . and thereby allow for their transformation or translation into useful meaning" (Grotstein, in Bion, 1993a, xiii). It is important to remember that for mother/infant and analyst/patient, much cannot be said in articulate language but instead must be intuited to result in a thinking couple.

Bion's concept of container is sometimes equated with Winnicott's idea of holding. However, the concepts have different qualities. The holding environment is "positive and growth promoting" (Symington & Symington, 1996, 58). Containment can be either positive or negative, although it is more often used in the positive meaning. Both the container and the contained are active in either integrative or destructive ways.

Next, we will discuss the K link, which Bion (1962) sees as "essentially a function of two objects, but it can be considered as a function of one" (p. 90), with the "earliest and most primitive manifestation of K occur [ring] in the relationship between mother and infant" (p. 90).

## The K Link

Believing that "an emotional experience cannot be conceived of in isolation from a relationship" (Bion, 1962, 42), Bion designates three factors – L (Love), H (Hate), and K (Knowledge) – to stand for the predominant link the patient establishes in the hour with the therapist. He sees any human as endlessly involved in establishing a link with another, but the linking might be most exquisitely loving or ragefully destructive. The "Knowledge" that Bion refers to as K is not static but more verb than noun, involving the effort to get to know and be receptive to what is true of an experience. Bion focused on the K link in psychoanalysis as it "is the link that is germane to learning by experience" (Bion, 1962: 47).

Bion's purpose in designating an L, H, or K link is, in thinking about an hour retrospectively, to get at what was most true of the emotional experience of the hour. The effort to grapple with the nature of the link could give a key to the communication:

> To sum up an emotional episode as K is to produce an imperfect record but a good starting point for the analyst's speculative meditation. In this regard the system I have sketched out, despite its crudity and naivety, possesses the rudiments of the essentials of a system of notation – record of fact and working tool.
>
> (Bion, 1962, 44)

If a child's desire to be known or to attack the possibility of being known seems predominant in an hour, then the K link would be the key to understanding his or her communication:

> The difference between the aim of the lie and the aim of truth can thus be expressed as a change of sense in x K y and to relate to intolerance of the pain associated with feelings of frustration.
>
> (Bion, 1962, 49)

If K appears predominant in a child's communication, then the type of K can be considered. Is the child trying to know herself or the object, or is the child too anxious to think about what goes on inside herself or another? If the child seems to be misunderstanding or denuding her experience, then the link is –K. If the child is expressing in his play a sense that he has no hope of a capacity to think, then the key to the hour is "no K." O'Shaughnessy (1988) describes "no K" as when the child is "expressing in his material a psychotic condition in which he exists without the capacity to think" (p. 182). Although Bion suggests that one mode of linking – L, H, or K – would predominate in a session, he means this in the service of thinking rather than in a formulaic manner. Bion followed Klein in seeing envy as the primary motivation for attacking the ability to think (–K), but other motivations to misunderstand can also be considered.

Here is a brief example of an hour that can be thought about in terms of the K link. Elizabeth was a brilliant 7-year-old girl who attended a school for gifted children. Her parents were highly successful professionals who divorced when Elizabeth was three. Her father, in particular, avoided emotions, which he chalked up to his British background. He was sent away to boarding school at 8. Elizabeth had started therapy six months earlier at the persistent urging of her school because of her emotional, relational, and behavioral problems. Although gifted, Elizabeth's emotional understanding lags far behind her intellectual capacities.

Elizabeth settled quickly into therapy after what seemed to her analyst to be an initial alertness to whether she would reject her. Soon after, the school reported behavioral, social, and emotional improvement. During the school year, her mother had brought Elizabeth regularly to her weekly therapy sessions. When summer came, father did not bring Elizabeth to therapy during the two weeks he had her. Although there was an agreement to reevaluate the therapy at six months, her father began raising concerns that therapy would go on "ad infinitum." His opposition to and withdrawal from therapy was concerning. Additionally, the analyst's two-week vacation also interfered with meetings. In total, five weeks of sessions were missed over the summer.

In the session after this gap, Elizabeth came in and wanted to play the board game *Sorry*, which she played in a highly competitive manner, conveying that winning was everything. The analyst felt aware of E.'s intelligence and sensed a no-win situation; the analyst would be a denigrated loser if she lost, and Elizabeth would be left with a feeling she wasn't ready for if she lost. Feeling uneasy about her own competitive feelings, the analyst commented on the competitive feeling and asked Elizabeth if she knew who was most competitive. Elizabeth said that she was. The analyst asked who was more competitive, Elizabeth's mom or her dad. She replied, "My dad." The analyst eventually won the game, and Elizabeth immediately claimed she had won and picked up the playing pieces about to throw them in the analyst's face.

To return to our concepts: these communications could be thought of as attacks on K. Elizabeth's knowledge of losing the game was attacked, as was the analyst, herself, as the winner of the game. But in a larger sense, there was an attack on any knowledge of loss or weakness. E.'s environment was not supporting her need for continuity, and this engendered a –K link in her. Unable to think at an emotional level, father and daughter could only think well on a purely intellectual basis. In this hour, Elizabeth was unable to compete and maintain an emotional connectedness simultaneously. Here, the –K was an effort not to know how full of rage she was at her parents and her analyst for not sustaining the opportunity for emotional connection. For Elizabeth to be able to have a K link, it would also have meant having to know things that were acutely painful. The break in the consistency of the therapy was but one of many links that had been broken in her life. Father did not want mother to have contact with Elizabeth when Elizabeth was with him, nor did he want to have contact with Elizabeth when she was with her mother. It is overwhelming for a child to know when a parent cannot be containing, and instead is breaking links out of anger. This had been a disruptive external feature of Elizabeth's childhood, so it was not surprising that links got broken inside of her. To generate a K link to her feelings about missing sessions would have brought Elizabeth close to knowledge of her father's emotional absence from her and of her parents' emotional absence from each other. A link to K could bring relief at understanding but also pain at having to know.

A flight into action (being about to throw the game pieces in the analyst's face) is not unusual in a young child whose internal resources are overwhelmed in relation to failures of containment. Bion describes –K in "the patient who appears to be unable to abstract, the patient to whom words are things – the things which the word is supposed to represent, but which are for him indistinguishable from their name and vice versa" (1962, 68–69). While a flight into action is far less out of step developmentally for a young child than for an adult, one could still describe this episode as –K. Bion saw all people as having psychotic aspects of their personality. While this child is only temporarily in a – K state, at this moment, she was "destroying rather than promoting knowledge" (1962, 98) as the envy and pain related to her losses were too much to tolerate.

Schneider, in an elaboration of Bion's concept of – K, comments on the "survival value of not knowing" (2005, 837). Schneider sees Bion as largely discussing – K in terms of envy but is aware that – K "goes far beyond envy as its only, or even its primary, motivating force" (p. 826). Schneider expands:

We all are destined to psychically kill our parents in the act of growing up (Loewald, 1979) and to harbor incestuous wishes. Fortunately, we are usually able not to know about such horrifying truths until we are sufficiently mature (as children or adults) and helped by our parents (or perhaps an analyst) to live with and make our peace with these human truths (along with other almost unbearable truths, such as the inescapability of our own death). Not knowing is, indeed, almost more important than knowing.

(p. 828)

## Transformation of "Beta" into "Alpha"

Bion coined the terms "alpha-elements" and "beta-elements" to designate fundamental mental experiences. He conceives of humans as endlessly transforming beta-elements (raw sensory data and unprocessed emotions) into alpha-elements (units of meaningful experience that can be thought, linked, and remembered), which he terms "alpha function." For Bion, dreaming is a paradigmatic of alpha function and goes on, not just in sleep, but all of the time. Bion sees the fundamental purpose of analysis as the patient's gain in alpha function through the analyst's maternal reverie and the pair's shared dreaming, which leads to the growth of the mind.

This view of dreaming sheds a particular light on play therapy. Ferro (1999) describes how various narrative derivatives are developed in child analysis through stories, play, drawing, dreaming, etc. Bion would see the play in play therapy as exactly right for the development of alpha function. Understandings of oneself are not generated in a linear manner but instead through the grasp of central narratives that are never static but constantly developing. This process is going on in both child and adult analysis. However, the playfulness of play therapy has a lot to lend to our treatment of adults. In *Attention and Interpretation*, Bion states:

Dream-like memory is the memory [memories that float into the mind unbidden] of psychic reality and is the stuff of analysis . . . the dream and the psycho-analyst's working material both share dream-like quality.

(1970, 70–71)

The play in play therapy allows the child a dream-like expression of her inner world and allows the analyst to participate in the meanings of the child's inner world that become shared meanings. In play therapy, we become interpreters of dreams in the form of play. Unmetabolized raw emotions, such as E.'s competitiveness and angry desire to throw the playing pieces in her analyst's face, are dreams in the hour. The analyst interprets dreams in the form of comments on and participation in the play. We will now consider these ideas in relation to a child in psychotherapy.

## Clinical Material

### History

Petite and slender with fair skin and short brown hair, Sydney (not her real name) began treatment when she was 9 years old, in the middle of third grade. Her parents expressed concern about Sydney's growing worries that she was "bad" at everything she tried to do, especially athletic and academic pursuits. Sydney's "bad" feelings also emerged in her dreams. She awoke frequently in the middle of the night, reporting nightmares about being taken away from her home. Terrified, she could only be consoled by snuggling with her mother for extended periods before being able to fall asleep again.

Sydney's capacity to know or to have a K link to something about her experiences was inconsistent at best. She would often burst into tears, unable to identify why she was feeling so upset. Likewise, Sydney's parents' ability to think about their daughter's developmental and emotional challenges also wavered. In the initial meeting with the therapist, Sydney's parents made brief mention of the fact that Sydney was a twin and that she and her sister were born prematurely from an IVF pregnancy. Sydney was diagnosed early on with cerebral palsy and had experienced multiple developmental delays. The parents' inability to discuss these complex beginnings revealed how painful it was for them to make a K link to them. The related anxieties had yet to be fully formulated or contained in the parents, never mind in Sydney.

Sydney's parents, both highly successful professionals, struggled for a number of years to begin a family. Sydney's mother was a first-generation Korean-American whose parents left the safety and comfort of their country to provide better opportunities for their children in the United States. In return, they expected their children to thrive and achieve, above all else, and to provide for future generations of family. Sydney's father was a fifth-generation Anglo-American from a prominent family who achieved enormous success in a number of business ventures. He had two sisters, both of whom had children early and easily.

Sydney's parents' failure to conceive naturally was especially painful and shameful to them, given their family histories. They underwent in-vitro fertilization procedures in their late thirties, resulting in Sydney's mother becoming pregnant with triplets. Fourteen weeks into her pregnancy, she experienced the loss of one of the fetuses. As Sydney's mother described this event, she rushed through the account as though wanting to provide the information but needed to move on quickly, leaving the therapist wondering more about her experience of this loss.

Sydney and her twin sister were born at 35 weeks. In contrast to her sister, who thrived and excelled, Sydney was delayed in meeting developmental milestones. She especially lagged in developing fine and gross motor skills, which affected her ability to walk in particular. At the age of 3 she was diagnosed with mild cerebral palsy and began attending occupational therapy, speech therapy, and physical therapy. Sydney attended her local public school, which was reputed to be one of the best in the area. When her struggles to learn became even more apparent, Sydney's parents moved her to an alternative school for children with learning disabilities.

Sydney initially enjoyed her new school. However, in the last several months, she has become more aware that she and her classmates are different in certain ways from other kids. Sydney's parents are reluctant to be more frank with Sydney about her learning and developmental challenges, fearing that she would feel stigmatized and incapable. As S.'s mother stated to the therapist, "In my family and in my culture, whatever challenges you have in life, no matter how hard, you face them and overcome them. I want S. to feel able to tackle her challenges, too." The challenge most apparent to Sydney's therapist was helping both her and her parents think about Sydney's growing awareness that she was different and that she struggled more than other children to speak, learn, think, and move. Not thinking about these differences, it seemed to the therapist, had left Sydney feeling that they were too hard to know (K) about.

Working with Sydney's parents proved to be challenging on many levels. Scheduling regular parent collateral meetings was difficult, given that the parents reported very busy schedules, including long periods in which Sydney's father traveled out of the country for his business dealings. When meetings were possible, S's mother prevailed over S's father in sharing her thoughts and concerns. She felt that she knew best what was happening for Sydney, given dad's frequent absences. The tension between Sydney's parents was palpable in these meetings. Sydney's mother appeared anxious or irritated when Sydney's father attempted to interject his observations or ideas. Sydney's father, in turn, would become irritated or defeated. Subtle projections of blame, insecurity, and ignorance from one parent to the other pervaded many of the initial meetings.

It seemed to Sydney's therapist that the parents were both anxious about Sydney and about their ability to parent her but were unable to provide support to one another. Sydney's therapist wondered about the parents' early experiences of containment from their own parents. Trying to help the parents think about their anxieties was a crucial step in working with Sydney's parents. In so doing, Sydney's therapist tried to create a space for the parents to come together as a strong couple who could allow for different perspectives in thinking about their daughter.

### Beginning Treatment

At first glance in the waiting room, Sydney's strained and cautious expression and her slow and stilted gait conveyed a palpable sense of uncertainty and unease. Her presentation changed dramatically over the course of the initial session and in subsequent sessions. A different side of Sydney emerged, revealing a range of powerful feelings – intense longing, painful frustration, and disturbing worry, to name a few. This shift in Sydney's affective presentation mirrors other oscillations in Sydney throughout the course of her treatment, including the shift in her ability to know (K) or not know (–K) about her experiences.

Bion's ideas about the importance of the therapist's capacity for maternal reverie and use of alpha function in transforming raw, unmetabolized emotions are particularly relevant in considering S.'s capacity to know something about herself with her therapist in two of her early sessions. In the first of these sessions, Sydney arrives in the company of two of her favorite dolls. Soft and beautiful, the Hapa dolls bear a striking resemblance to Sydney.[3]

As she brings her dolls into the consulting room, Sydney giggles, telling the therapist, with a sparkle in her eyes, that her babies have some worries they want to discuss with her – but only after the therapist and Sydney play a game.

Painstakingly, Sydney sets up a game of Mancala.[4] Though Sydney's coordination makes it difficult for her to place the marbles correctly in their places, she does so, announcing that she will go first. As Sydney proceeds through her turn with great determination and growing excitement, she whispers under her breath and mumbled something that is barely audible. Leaning in closer, the therapist finally makes out the words: "I'm going to win, I'm going to win, I'm going to win!" Sydney spoke softly but fiercely. When her turn is technically over, Sydney continues playing, skipping over her therapist's turn several times so she can accumulate more marbles, continuing to whisper her mantra, "I'm going to win." Her therapist responds, "You want so much to win. It feels so good to win and so hard to lose." Sydney's therapist has an awful feeling of impending defeat. Sydney proceeds to pass her by in the game, shrieking with delight with each additional marble gained. Sydney ultimately wins the game, leaving her therapist with an unexpected experience of great, inevitable loss.

At this point in the session, something shifted in Sydney. The unmetabolized emotion she had experienced in relation to her great fear of defeat had been taken in and contained by her therapist. The therapist's use of alpha function to describe the defeat allowed her to development to occur, expressed in the next sequence of the session.

Setting aside the Mancala game, Sydney looks over at her dolls and then looks back at the therapist and smiles.

T:  What do your friends think of being here?
S:  They like coming here. They like being able to talk about their worries.
T:  Do you think they have any worries to tell me about?
S:  They do. But they want to tell you about them later.
T:  Maybe it's a little hard for them to talk about what they're worried about.
S:  (Whispers to her doll and pretends to listen to her doll whispering back.)

*T:* What did she say?

*S:* She's afraid a stranger will come and take her away from home. She's pretty worried, but it helps to have her other baby friend around with her.

*T:* She feels safer when she knows others are there.

*S:* Yes. And there's something else, too. She gets worried because she doesn't know how to talk as well as some other kids at school. She's afraid she's going to get made fun of by the bullies at school. They don't understand that she can't help the way she talks.

*T:* You're thinking of how sad it would feel to be teased. I wonder if we can ask your friend how she feels about it.

*S:* She wants to tell you herself. But she wants to whisper it.

*T:* Maybe it's hard to talk about. (The therapist leans over to hear the doll's whispers) Aha .... Mmmm .... Aha .... Oooh.

*S:* What did she say?

*T:* She says it feels really bad to be teased. And she worries about why she talks differently from the other kids.

*S:* Well, why does she? (S. gets up and lies next to her doll. She nestles into the doll's body and looks up at the therapist.)

*T:* You know, I think some people ... they're just born a little differently, and the way they walk and talk can be different, too. But it's hard when other people don't understand that.

*S:* I think my friend likes coming here. I think she's going to want to come next time, too.

In the second part of the hour, through the therapist's maternal reverie related to fears about being different, unwanted, and misunderstood, a transformation occurred. A K link was established between Sydney and her therapist, and the beta elements were processed through the therapist's alpha function. The end result was that Sydney was able to experience the desire and capacity to think about herself.

### From K to −K

The following session with Sydney begins very differently, with an initial disruption.

*S:* arrives 15 minutes late. Her mother, harried and breathless, explained that the counselors at Sydney's camp had forgotten that she had to leave early for her appointment. As Sydney enters the consulting room, she smiles wearily at her therapist, asking in a deflated tone if they will have less time together. The therapist acknowledges that their time will be shorter because someone at camp had gotten confused. "It was a mistake," Sydney says gravely to her therapist. Sydney also reports that she forgot to bring her doll friends with her. Faced with the prospect of having so much less today, Sydney sighs and suggests they play Mancala.

*S.* announces that she gets to go first because she is always the winner – the "pro" – and the therapist is always the "loser." S. also insists on playing by her rules, which includes taking as many turns as she likes. Once again, the therapist feels left out of the game, hopeless, and defeated. When the therapist lets S. know that it feels bad to never have a turn, S. begins very quietly to hum a tune, compelling the therapist to lean in closer to hear what she is saying.

*S:* What? Why are you looking at me?

*T:* I thought I heard you singing something. But I wasn't sure. I guess I'm curious about what you might be singing.

*S:* It's the winners' song. But only winners know it.

*T:* I see. Boy, it's funny to be able to almost hear it but not be able to make it out. It makes me feel like I'm not really a winner.

*S:* You can be, though. It just takes practice. Lots and lots of practice. Like practice almost all the time.

*T:* That sounds like a lot of work.

*S:* It is.

*T:* What if I work really hard and still don't get it?

*S:* You will.

*T:* It just feels hard now not to win.

*S:* Yeah, it does.

*T:* It sounds like you understand.

In this sequence, the therapist once again absorbed Sydney's loser, outwitted feelings, allowing them to begin to understand something together. S. conveyed a sense of wanting to be able to do what her therapist could do – to use alpha function to make sense of previously unintegrated emotions (beta elements).

Sydney then proceeds to take her therapist's seat, literally, by moving over to her therapist's chair and sprawling across it, her feet hanging over the edge. Sydney stretches one of her feet toward the therapist, who is still sitting on the ground and touches the therapist's shoe. Sydney gazes at the shoe and then suddenly becomes aware that she has encountered something new. She wonders aloud, "What's that?" When the therapist points out that it was her shoe, Sydney erupts in giggles and says softly, "Our feet are touching. They're connecting." Sydney proceeds to touch the therapist's hands, one by one, with her hands. She rests for a moment, hands and feet connecting, gazing down at the therapist. The therapist has an image (i.e., a maternal reverie) of two babies encountering one another in the womb.

This reverie is disrupted, however, when Sydney remembers that she and her therapist would miss a session when Sydney was away on vacation the following week. Sydney felt bad and noticed something "bad" on the therapist's desk as well: a diet soda.

*S:* You shouldn't drink that. My mom told me. It's not healthy, and you'll get fat.

*T:* What would happen if I got fat?

*S:*  Well, probably you would get so big that you won't be able to get into your car.

*T:*  So I won't be able to go certain places.

*S:*  And if you get really fat, you won't be able to go into your house. Your big, fat butt will get stuck in the doorway.

*T:*  So I won't be able to go home if I don't take care of myself.

*S:*  (Getting up to throw the cup away) There! Don't drink anymore. If you do, I'm going to put a sign up in your office that says, "The worry doctor is fat!" And then everyone will know.

After experiencing closeness, expressed by the physical contact she and her therapist had with one another, Sydney became anxious that the time with her therapist must come to an end. The "bad" soda evoked a third object for Sydney, representing the therapist's link with other experiences and relationships apart from Sydney. Unable to think about something that separates her from her therapist, Sydney attacks the link between herself and her therapist (–K), discarding the drink – and, along with it, an experience of knowledge (K) and potential containment of the pain of separation and envy or jealousy.

## Discussion

The first hour between Sydney and her therapist demonstrated that once the therapist acknowledged Sydney's joy at victory and tolerated her own miserable defeat, then a softer process emerged. They were able to play with the dolls through an imaginary conversation that showed them dreaming together in a way that characterized the use of alpha function. Their back-and-forth imaginary dialogue illustrated not only how K is nurtured through this kind of play but also how it became an instrument for internalizing therapeutic containment. After the therapist verbalized an understanding of the projective identification of loser, a K link emerged around the ways in which Sydney felt different (bullied, how she talks, her fear of losing her parents). Feeling diminished and inferior are vulnerable areas for Sydney that cloud her fragile tolerance for thinking how she is different from her peers.

The second hour, on the other hand, shows that when holding fails – as in the late arrival and the surprise of the upcoming missed appointment – then there is little place for K to sustain itself. We might, therefore, consider that in some circumstances, holding is a necessary primary condition in order for containing to persist and not collapse. This session is full of –K, since Sydney feels persecuted by the events that produced the failure of holding her psychologically. Initially, she punishes her therapist with another lesson in hardness since one must "practice all the time" to gain the glory of the "winner's song." The therapist handles this well enough, and, as a result, something between them rights itself during a moment of unanticipated physical contact that allows for softened exposure of giggles, touch, and delight.

Unfortunately, this moment cannot be sustained, and it is interesting to ponder what interferes with it. The therapist's reverie perhaps provides a bit of a clue since, in this, she imagines that they are two babies in a womb. It seems that this image evokes aspects of what is consciously missing for Sydney about her origins – that she arrived into the world as a very complicated baby and developed quite differently from her sibling. Within this reverie, the therapist might also be representing an elusive sense of the losses that occurred during the pregnancy and around the realization of Sydney's own difficulties upon birth. Although speculative, the therapist, through her imagination, is functioning here like a mother who "sees" in her mind all her babies. This representation potentially reaches deep into a part of Sydney's "reality" that she is unaware of, a reality of loss, secrecy, and traumatic birth. Aside from this, it touches upon Sydney's psychic reality of what she imagines happened to her to make her different. Perhaps the therapist's reverie may point to a kind of K link for which Sydney is not yet prepared because it is so complex. At this point, the physical touching may have been too much, and it overwhelmed Sydney with feelings of her own soft baby self, which in her mind has to be dealt with harshly to blot out any recognition of her differences.

Suddenly, Sydney directs her attention to the "bad" soda that will damage her therapist. This paranoid attack appears precipitated by a fantasy of a "fat" therapist, one whose fatness might mean pregnancy. In this unconscious tangle, Sydney acts out that the waste must be got rid of when she throws the cup into the garbage. Could this cup stand in some encrypted, hidden way for loss and difference that date to Sydney's birth? The supposed fatness of the therapist becomes, for Sydney, a way to imagine her therapist as persecuted by an impressive difference that everyone will be able to see. At the end of the session, because of Sydney's extreme feelings of persecution and vulnerability, she seems temporarily both unheld and uncontained, and attacks on any potential K link predominate.

In his collection *Second Thoughts,* Bion writes about "The imaginary twin" (1993b, 3–22). In this paper, Bion states, "The function of the imaginary twin was thus to deny a reality different from himself" (p. 19). Bion describes this as part of the transference that an adult man establishes toward him, a transference that feels rigid and scripted to Bion. The practical effect of this situation is that it encumbers the patient's tolerance for any "internal psychic reality" (p. 19), resulting in an obliteration of differences. Sydney's domination of her therapist likewise is in service of seeking to control her because she dreads that the therapist could make her aware of being different and facing the feelings associated with it, i.e., in Sydney's fantasy, she would be like a loser.

When Sydney subjects her therapist to playing by rigid rules, she diminishes the possibility of the therapist's freedom to play either cooperatively or competitively. Knowledge is thereby limited for both of them because Sydney's projective identifications require her therapist to take on the loser identity. Sydney's control of the therapist functions psychologically to limit the emergence of any K link. Unfortunately, for a child of 9 with a developmental disability, such defensiveness can impede the growth of her mind and undermine what she is actually capable of.

We might wonder here about the history that Sydney does not know, namely her conception through IVF. Certainly, her prenatal history was complicated by the lost triplet. With multiple in-vitro fertilization (IVF), there is a 10% chance of a "vanishing twin," a statistic that has been confirmed repeatedly and now has led to guidelines advising implantation of a single embryo (Pinborg et al., 2005; Sazonova et al., 2011). In addition, there is an increased risk with multiple IVF of cerebral palsy and other neurological impairments in the surviving fetus when one has vanished (Anand et al., 2007). Given that Sydney was conceived through IVF over ten years ago, her parents made the best decision they thought possible at that time. Although this area of medical research has evolved rapidly, we might wonder how the *in utero* loss affected Sydney's parents. In particular, a complex web of loss shaped Sydney's entry into the world. Is it remotely possible that she carried from her prenatal development an unconscious imprint of a lost other, the vanished triplet? While there is no way to know for sure, Sydney did share her mother's experience of loss, and this likely affected the infant-mother relationship.

Early on, Sydney's mother commented to the therapist that she believed in overcoming hard challenges, no matter what. Might that be an attitude that was too hard by many degrees for a child such as Sydney? Indeed, hardness was inflicted on her therapist when the rules were arbitrarily changed to ensure the therapist's consistent defeat. In contrast, Sydney's need for softer nurturance was evident through many aspects of the sessions, including the arrival of the dolls and, more importantly, her desire for physical contact with her therapist. In these interactions, Sydney's need for holding, as articulated by Winnicott, and containing from her therapist come to the fore. Ogden has commented on the different qualities of these functions as follows: holding is centered on guaranteeing the child's experience of "being and becoming over time," whereas containing involves the emergence of a capacity for alpha function in which container and contained are "in tension" (Ogden, 2004b, 1362). Holding, in other words, supports the environmental factors that enable K, and containing optimally leads to the actualization of K within a relationship.

Sydney's parents had not spoken with her about the difficulties during the pregnancy. While they were rightfully cautious about overwhelming her with too much information, the case raises interesting questions. How is IVF incorporated or not into a child's origin story? Does it even need to have a place in it? We have only to think of Freud's "Remembering, repeating, and working through" (1914) or Fraiberg's "Ghosts in the nursery" (1975) to hypothesize that children can infer much about what is not spoken, discussed, or acknowledged. Particularly salient, as Sydney's case shows us, is that the "reality" of her story, of how she came into this world, derives from the background of her conception through IVF and her subsequent fetal development. How does K fit into this sort of story, especially since Sydney was struggling with her differences? She would most likely turn to her parents for answers, and of course, she would further develop fantasies of her own about her origins.

A true K link is not just about the "reality" of a medical record, but rather it pertains to an ability to know one's differences and share them with a receptive other. Perhaps a problem with parents using IVF could be tentativeness or heightened anxiety about naming differences out of fear that the "reality" could be too hurtful, overwhelming, and unpleasant. A child therapist always has to watch for parental communications that reinforce an idea that it is better not to know certain things because a child might stretch this to include aspects of knowledge about herself, aspects that may or may not have all that much to do with "reality." Psychic reality, of course, includes unconscious fantasies, memories, emotions, thoughts, and other motivations for behaviors.

Freud (1914) makes the point that forgetting an experience and never having been aware of something are two different aspects of not knowing. He nonetheless finds,

> As regards the course taken by psychical events it seems to make no difference whatever whether such a "thought-connection" was conscious and then forgotten or whether it never managed to become conscious at all.
>
> (Freud, 1914, 149)

In other words, an unconscious "thought-connection" suffices to set in motion a painful repetition that is attempting to force upon the conscious psyche an awareness of something hidden. Prior consciousness is not a prerequisite. In this regard, Sydney's parents, and many other parents, too, may place a greater value on not knowing as protective and shielding from a truth that they consider too much for the child to bear. We also have to wonder: for whom is it too much? Unfortunately, this attitude would seem to undermine the value of K links. Bion's contributions of K (and –K), as well as attacks on linking, may add to understanding circumstances, especially those of loss when a child or adolescent repeats certain behaviors because she wants to know more fully her story, but has been "protected" from it far too long. Absent this analytic recognition, a child might otherwise persist in protecting herself from knowing her own internal world with its oedipal fantasies about her parents, her birth, and how she came to be. That would be a further loss.

Too frequently, parents hide losses from their children. In Sydney's case, there are several losses: the parents' own struggle with fertility, the vanished triplet, and Sydney's disability with the differences it brings for her. It may be that because of the first, her parents have decided not to tell her about the second, but more importantly, not to openly converse with her about the third. With the increasing use of medically assisted technologies for fertilization, more children are being born who have very complicated and challenging stories about their origins. Parents sometimes ignore these, hoping that "ignorance is bliss." At other times, they err by overloading a child with scientific details that cannot be processed by a tender, young mind. For example, a 6-year-old boy with a history of IVF via an anonymous sperm donor told one of us that he knew he came "from the fridge" and that he believed his father to be someone named "Don't know" (the boy's misinterpretation of the word "donor"). In such cases, a dependable creation story that the child can own as his or hers is missing – one that the child can play with, dream about, and share with others. We can see in Sydney's case that she struggles mightily with what she can know of herself – that she is different from other children in many ways that hurt and that she might wish were not so. Her therapist's interventions during the doll play of the first hour opened the door to thinking about herself and her differences. The fragility of this gain toward K is made apparent by the –K states that prevail in the second hour.

This case brings up some of the new, complex dynamics surrounding the growing field of fertility treatments. Child psychotherapists and analysts working with families who use assisted reproductive technology will continue to have their work cut out for them in advising parents how not to rely on an attitude of not knowing when some greater tolerance for K could go a long way toward easing a child's anxiety about exploring for herself the question "who am I?" We might agree with Bion (2005) that the problem is not with children's unmyelinated nerve fibers but rather with their parents' myelinated ones that have become a bit too impermeable.[5] This may be where a major conflict around the value of K is waged and where a defensive avoidance of K can be addressed therapeutically.

## Notes

1  As is well known, Klein was Bion's second analyst. Klein cited her analysis of young children as the most fundamental source of her thinking.
2  Bion uses "mother" to refer to the infant's primary object; it could equally be a father.
3  "Hapa" is a Hawaiian word, borrowed from the English word "half," used to describe people of mixed Asian or Pacific Island descent, including people who are half Asian and half Caucasian.
4  In the game of Mancala, players collect piles of marbles distributed along a game board and deposit them in a container, or Mancala, at the end of the board. The player who collects the most marbles in her Mancala wins.
5  See Brady (2011) for a Bionian approach to working with parents.

## References

Anand, D., Platt, M.J., & Pharoah, P.O. (2007). Vanishing twin: A possible cause of cerebral impairment. *Twin Research and Human Genetics*, 10, 202–209.

Bion, W.R. (1962). *Learning from Experience*. London: Karnac.

Bion, W.R. (1970). Attention and interpretation. In *Seven Servants*. New York: Jason Aronson.

Bion, W.R. (1993a). *Second Thoughts: Selected Papers on Psychoanalysis*. New York: Jason Aronson.

Bion, W.R. (1993b). The imaginary twin. In *Second Thoughts: Selected Papers on Psychoanalysis* (pp. 3–22). New York: Jason Aronson.

Bion, W.R. (2005). *The Tavistock Seminars*. London: Karnac.

Brady, M.T. (2011). The individual in the group: An application of Bion's group theory to parent work in child analysis and child psychotherapy. *Contemporary Psychoanalysis*, 47(3), 420–437.

Brown, L. (2012). Bion's discovery of Alpha function: Thinking under fire on the battlefield and in the consulting room. *International Journal of Psychoanalysis*, 93, 1191–1214.

Ferro, A. (1999). *The Bi-Personal Field: Explorations in Child Analysis*. London: Routledge.

Fraiberg, S., Adelson, E., & Shapiro, V. (1975). Ghosts in the nursery: A psychoanalytic approach to the problems of impaired infant-mother relationships. *Journal of the American Academy of Child Psychiatry*, 14, 387–421.

Freud, S. (1914). Remembering, repeating and working through. *SE*, 12, 147–156.

Klein, M. (1975). Notes on some schizoid mechanisms. In *Envy and Gratitude*. London: The Hogarth Press. (Original work published 1946.)

Loewald, H. (1979). The waning of the Oedipus complex. In *Papers on Psychoanalysis* (pp. 384–404). New Haven, CT: Yale University Press.

Ogden, T.H. (2004a). An introduction to the reading of Bion. *International Journal of Psychoanalysis*, 85, 285–300.

Ogden, T.H. (2004b). On holding and containing, being and dreaming. *International Journal of Psychoanalysis*, 85, 1349–1364.

O'Shaughnessy, E. (1988). W.R. Bion's theory of thinking and new techniques in child analysis. In E. Bott-Spillius (Ed.), *Melanie Klein Today: Developments in Theory and Practice, Volume I: Mainly Theory* (pp. 177–190). London: Routledge.

Pinborg, A., Lidegaard, O., La Cour Freiesleben, N., & Andersen, A.N. (2005). Consequences of vanishing twins in IVF/ICSI pregnancies. *Human Reproduction*, 20, 2821–2829.

Sazonova, A., Källen, K., Thurin-Kjellberg, A., Wennerholm., U.B., & Bergh, C. (2011). Factors affecting obstetric outcome of singletons born after IVF. *Human Reproduction*, 26(10), 2878–2886. http://doi.org/10.1093/humrep/der241.

Schneider, J.A. (2005). Experiences in K and – K. *International Journal of Psychoanalysis*, 86, 825–839.

Symington, J., & Symington, N. (1996). *The Clinical Thinking of Wilfred Bion*. New York, NY: Routledge.

# Chapter 7

# Considerations Regarding the Establishment of Play Space

## Shifting Psychic States in a 5-Year-Old

Winnicott places playing at the heart of psychoanalytic treatment:

> Psychotherapy takes place in the overlap of two areas of playing, that of the patient and that of the therapist. Psychotherapy has to do with two people playing together. The corollary of this is that where playing is not possible then the work done by the therapist is directed towards bringing the patient from a state of not being able to play into a state of being able to play.
>
> (1971, 38)

In a similar vein, Winnicott sees play as universal and psychoanalysis as "a highly specialized form of playing in the service of communicating with oneself and others" (1971, 41). The transitional phenomena of infancy (in whatever rich, barren or traumatized form) lead to the capacity to play and on into the intermediate space of cultural experience (Winnicott, 1953, 1971). Likewise, as Elise (2018) suggests, analytic process transforms painful affect not mainly by naming but through the enlivening experience of creating, which in itself promotes healing.

But how is a play space established when a child is trapped in a nightmare state of mind or in rigid, repetitive defenses? In this paper, I would like to explore three shifting states in a small patient of mine: perseverative action, play space and nightmare world. I saw my work in the hour I will relate as an effort to create a play space, which seemed constantly at risk of collapsing into either perseverative action or overwhelming waking nightmare. I agree with Mayes and Cohen (1993) that "the very process of enactment through fantasy play in the space of the analysis is, in and of itself, developmentally restorative" (1236). Winnicott saw the experience of play and the use of illusion (in its healthy sense)[1] as what allows us to feel alive. I will use this boy's shifting states to try to consider aspects relevant to what makes a child able to play. I will add some considerations regarding the facilitation of this 'highly specialized form of playing' in adults.

Parsons's description of the analyst's "paradoxical state of mind" (2000) in approaching the intermediate space of psychoanalysis is relevant to creating a play space. The paradoxical state of mind Parsons conveys is that of "waiting properly" (2000). That is, in Parsons' view, waiting properly in analysis requires openness to

DOI: 10.4324/9781003498810-8

catching spontaneously occurring unconscious processes in our patients and in us while simultaneously listening in a very rigorous, complex manner. This waiting also requires some tolerance for experiences of deadness in the analytic space. In the surfing metaphor of this book, the analyst needs to be able to wait to catch the wave that will allow something to happen.

With children, play is the equivalent of free association. I would suggest the reverse captures the truth better – in adults, free association is the equivalent of play. What is important about playing and verbal associations is not just the communication of psychic contents but also the intermediate nature of the experience. No one asks the small child if the blanket is really his mother – it is and it isn't. Likewise, in analysis, we try to grow the imaginary space where experiences of self and others can be played with. Play does not just convey emotion and unconscious phantasy but develops the child's imaginary resources to deal with emotions and phantasy. Also, as Anderson says, "[C]hildren have not yet managed to apply the bandages that adults protect themselves with – 'adulthood,' 'intellectualization,' 'cooperation,' 'being a good patient'" (1997, 425). The freest of free association in adults may not have quite the raw quality that Anderson describes: "a child in a playroom constantly on the move, now playing, now with toys, now role-playing, now trying to get me to act, now talking thoughtfully to me" (1997, 425). But Anderson here seems to be describing a child largely in a state of play.

To consider the establishment or collapse of play space, I will describe the ebb and flow from a perseverative repetitive non-play to play space to a nightmare world in a session with a 5-year-old patient.

## 'Justin'

### History

Justin's parents came to me when he was 5 for a series of consultations. They described him as anxious and prone to shame. He would knock his head against the wall and say, "Bad Justin." Mother had a high-risk pregnancy due to early cervical changes and then had an emergency C-section. Justin has two older sisters, neither of whom has evidenced significant problems. Justin's parents described him as having been a fussy, colicky baby and as "cognitively restless." Justin's parents expressed concern that he was frequently pushed out of the way by other children at his academically oriented pre-kindergarten. In these situations, he seemed frozen and unable to speak up for himself.

From infancy, Justin was overwhelmed by any loud sound or commotion. He would collapse in distress at noises other children might not be bothered by. To make matters worse, from ages 9 months to 2 years, Justin had a series of illnesses and intrusive diagnostic procedures. He had high fevers and febrile seizures with respiratory viruses and meningitis. His scientist father broke into sobs, describing how Justin had awoken from sleep terrified during a lumbar puncture. Father described having to hold Justin down during the lumbar puncture while Justin fought "like a tiger." "Vials and vials" of blood were drawn from Justin, his chest was X-rayed and he was catheterized during various procedures. His illness had completely resolved, and since this difficult period, Justin has been in good physical health.

Justin's mother related struggling with significant anxiety, both in relation to her childhood and particularly during Justin's illnesses. What stood out most about her childhood was her retelling of her mother's multiple miscarriages. She recalled seeing the bloody bathroom as her mother was rushed to the hospital after a miscarriage. Such incidents would never be spoken of in the family after they happened, leaving her alone and frozen in her fears.

In contrast to mother's anxiety about Justin, father seemed to minimize Justin's problems. His own parents had divorced when he was 3, and his parents subsequently lived far apart so that he only saw his father occasionally. He had longed to be a father, but he wanted a far less anxious son than Justin, with whom he could enjoy rough and tumble father-son times.

## Beginning Treatment

After three months of meeting with the parents, I recommended that I should meet with Justin. I made this recommendation when the parents reported that Justin was immobilized by fear at his pre-kindergarten. His fear had worsened after another boy bit him badly, which Justin, frozen, had not even protested. This preliminary period of parent work seemed to help to establish some beginning trust from his parents in me and a sense that we would continue to collaborate on Justin's behalf.

Justin is a handsome, angelic-looking child. He still has a trace of the baby to him while also solidly looking like a little boy. During our first session, I was struck by Justin's verbal precocity. I watched his lips struggle to form the word 'obelisk.' I had the impression that his body could not keep up with the speed of his mind, leaving him frustrated.

During this first session, I asked Justin: "If you had three wishes, what would they be?" He at first said that was "tricky," and I thought he might not answer. Then he said, "I wish I was a snake so then I could be underground where the mice are, but the lions aren't." Later, I showed him the Squiggle game (Winnicott, 1971). He made of my squiggle: "A snake with a mouse. He can smell with his tongue, and his eyes can see heat, blood." This play led me to think that Justin lived in a psychic world filled with fear of violent aggression, which he tried to handle by staying out of sight. I was struck by his intelligence in creating a story that so well represented his fears and his ways of defending himself. While Justin had seemed anxious leaving his father to come into the room with me, I thought he responded well to the offer of a play space. I spoke with his parents about his need to have a space to play out his fears, and they accepted a three-times-a-week schedule.

While well-behaved at school, in his sessions with me, Justin was soon noisy, with frequent loud crashes and jumping from the furniture onto the floor. I often felt startled by the crashes. As he settled into treatment, he often called me a "dumb-dumb" or a "booty face." He told me, "I am going to kick your butt." When returned to his mother at the end of a session, he would hug her and then stick his shoes in her face. I thought he was trying to be aggressive with the people he felt it was safest to experiment with and not have to stay solely underground or frozen. He was never actually physically rough with me at this point, so his aggression was not truly alarming. I imagined that *he* would feel alarmed if he got physical with me and that playing out violent or aggressive stories at a distance was of relief to him. This reminded me of Winnicott's sense of the importance of aggression as a part of aliveness.

At times, Justin seemed more disorganized and overwhelmed. One day, Justin arrived at a session after a teacher had lost his jacket at school. In his session, Justin said to me, "You have to smell the trash, and you have blood on your face." I felt distressed and alarmed by his visceral descriptions of my body coming apart. His experience of feeling lost track of by his teacher seemed to lead to overwhelming feelings of bodily anxiety and disintegration. I reflected on Didier Anzieu's (2016/1985) conception of ruptures of the skin ego experienced as the subjective sense of coming apart,[2] which for Justin likely was linked to his early medical intrusions. In other words, the loss of the coat was not of a prized and comforting object, but much more literally the loss of something that made him feel like he was held together in a skin-coat. At times, Justin could actually tell me about fears – of homeless people or seeing a man without a leg. This fear of the loss of a home-coat likewise had the terror quality of dissolving without a house-skin or body parts being ripped off.

Justin's play became occupied with themes of puncture, teeth, blood and skeletons. He played out being dead over and over. I asked him, "Do you feel afraid you might die?" He said, "Yes." I talked to him about trauma, saying: "When something too big has happened to us, it stays inside us in an undigested way, and it can feel like it is still happening to us now, even though it isn't." He seemed to calm down after my comment, and I felt he had understood what I said.

I thought that Justin's experience of febrile seizures was represented in his current jarring experiences of dissociation and discontinuity. Mother had told me that there had been times when Justin's fever was so high that he talked as if he was another person. I thought that experiences of being delusional with fever and 'not himself' when ill were finding a way into the hour. In the play, he frequently shot me, but in a disturbing way that had the quality of my body coming apart. "I shot off your lips, your eye; there is blood coming down." Justin spoke reluctantly about frequent nightmares, such as of his arm being cut off or someone who was not his mommy pretending she was his mommy. These descriptions were brief, as he quickly became overwhelmed with fear as he told me a nightmare.

### Clinical Material

I will offer an extended vignette to consider Justin's different psychic states. At the time of the session, Justin had been in analysis with me for six months. In this session, he came readily to my office:

*J:*   So, what were we doing? (He frequently asks me to write down where we are leaving off when we end a session and then asks me if I remember what we were doing last time as we start.)

*T:*   You like to pick up right where we left off – you asked me to write it down.

*J:*   (Somewhat impatiently) I don't need it. I remember. You were going to be in the bad guy fortress. (In this play, I am a bad guy and am persistently killed or captured by Justin, the head of the good guys. I have been allowed one bad guy friend, Jeff, who is also captured.) You are tied up, and Jeff is a giant. He tries to escape and he is shot through the eye and dies.

*T:*   Oh no, Jeff is dead and now I am alone in the Bad Guy Fortress. (I am supposed to be tied up, so I have my arms crossed. I am sitting on the floor to equalize our heights. Justin is running around with two guns, shooting at me. This part of the play goes on for several minutes. Eventually, I remind Justin that we are going to talk or draw after we play for ten minutes. More shooting. At one point, Justin crashes down to the floor and pretends to be dead.)

*T:*   Are you dead? Oh no! Justin is dead.

*J:*   You're a bad guy; don't ask about me.

*T:*   Okay, I wonder what happens when someone dies?

*J:*   (Gets up) I'm half human, half robot. (Justin does some mechanical moves and jumps off the armchair loudly.)

*T:*   You like crashes.

*J:*   No, I don't. (More shooting and one giant crash, jumping off the chair).

*T:*   Okay, that's too loud for downstairs.

*J:*   No, it's not.

*T:*   We need to do our talking or check on Inferno (a monster he has been drawing).

*J:*   No.

*T:*   It's been ten minutes, it's time. (I open his folder of drawings and he sits down.)

*J:*   I'm going to draw me as half robot. (He proceeds to draw two figures. One is his outside, which looks like a person, and his inside, which is a robot – mechanical looking.)

*T:*   How can you tell if it's human or robot?

*J:*   The way you can tell if it's a robot is it shoots lasers out its eyes. It has some mechanical part that protrudes outside the human part, but which can be retracted. It also has invisible buttons on its leg to push the mechanical part up and down. (He writes down the code that you need to know to kill the robot. He draws lasers that emerge from the robot's eyes.) The lasers stay inside the rings, or they would be out of control.

*T:*   Is it scary?

*J:*  I wouldn't be scared because the lasers are coming out of my eyes.

*T:*  So, I'd be scared because I could see the lasers.
(Justin draws a machine inside the robot that has waves that remind me of a heart monitor.)

*T:*  Those waves remind me of machines in the hospital that record your heart rate. (Justin doesn't respond.)

*J:*  Is it ten minutes yet?

*T:*  Not quite.

*J:*  (Drawing) These are earpieces that allow the robot to amplify sound.

*T:*  Does a robot really want to hear what other people say? I guess humans are curious, like if we want to hear what someone is whispering, but I don't know about robots.

*J:*  Well, I'd want to know if someone is trying to kill me.

*T:*  I was thinking of how you were afraid you were going to die, or maybe it's like you feel a part of you did die – like a part of you is now robot. (He doesn't respond verbally, but I feel that he has registered what I've said.)

*J:*  I'm going to draw my monster. (It has several eyes with 'angry' eyebrows. It has many sharp teeth. It also has one very long tooth that is hidden. He draws a monster for me but says it is a giant; it has smaller teeth than his monster and only one that is sharp. He gives it a snake for hair and says):

*J:*  It's not like Medusa because the snake is in the hair. (He draws three heads on my monster. Something about the inhuman part of this sequence has left me with an ominous feeling.)
(At this point, I mention an upcoming disruption in sessions we will have. He tells me that they will be in Flo*rida.)*

*J:*  It was my birthday on Saturday (he sounds disappointed).

*T:*  Did you want to have a party? (His parents have told me he can be immobilized at parties.)

*J:*  Not a big one.

*T:*  I wonder if it was hard for you and your parents to know what you wanted, but then it was kind of disappointing. (He is still drawing teeth.)

*T:*  Your drawing makes me think of the boy that bit you. (He doesn't respond.)

*T:*  Have you lost any teeth yet?

*J:*  No, but one is wiggly.

*J:*  What's that like?

*J:*  (He looks uncomfortable.) But you get money.

*T:*  It's so normal to lose a tooth. Your bigger teeth are growing in and need the room but it can feel so strange to lose a part of yourself you've always had. Maybe that was making you feel worried you could lose another body part, like your arm.

*J:*  Do you know Megan?

*T:*  No, is she in your class?

*J:*  Yes, she lost two teeth, and they put them in this small green box.

*T:*  It sounds like it feels exciting to lose a tooth, too.

I will end my vignette here, close to the end of the hour.

I noticed that I was somewhat playful in this hour but guardedly so. I think this has to do with my fear for Justin in this session. Likewise, Justin's psychic space for playfulness is limited, as mental states collapse into either too terrifying or too repetitive. In other words, a nightmare or a perseverative world is not a play world. I struggled at times with the repetitive nature of some of Justin's play. The word 'perseverative' came to my mind as stronger than the more commonly used 'stuck' or 'repetitive' play. Merriam-Webster defines 'perseverative' as "continuation of something (such as repetition of a word) usually to an exceptional degree or beyond a desired point." I came to feel that Justin needed a limit placed on his perseverative play in order to draw him toward a potential space for more interactive, imaginative play.

Alvarez suggests that a therapist may need to "interrupt the (seemingly but falsely playful) playing child or over-chatty adolescent to convey our own demand for, and insistence on, a more real meaning" (2012, 156). Similarly, Rhode, in her Foreword to the new edition of Tustin's *Autistic States in Children* (2021/1992), notes that Tustin saw "autistic self-protective strategies as part of the human condition – tragically restrictive, though felt to be necessary" (xvii). I am reminded that Tustin insisted that autistic children say hello and goodbye at the beginning and end of the session – not as a behavioral intervention to get them to seem more 'normal' but rather to insist that *she was there* so that gradually she might dawn on them as someone worth knowing.

### Discussion

I would like to 'play' with this vignette by dividing it up into three segments. The first is *Crashes and Boundaries*; the second is *Robots and Fear of Psychosis*; and the third is *Teeth and the Ebb and Flow of the Healthy and the Disturbed*.

#### Crashes and Boundaries

In the first part of the hour (Crashes and Boundaries), Justin's good guy/bad guy play feels somewhat communicative to me, but it also feels flat. I can see that he wants me to be the one who is fearful and helpless. This needs room, but I also have the sense it is not really going anywhere. I have had a similar sense in prior sessions, so I have told him we need to have some time to talk and draw. Here, I am trying to wait properly (Parsons, 2000) but also to know when more waiting may not be in order. Drawing and talking more directly about fears have seemed like more fertile ground in Justin's hours. Secondly, my long-suffering downstairs analyst neighbor has complained to me about the crashes during Justin's hours. I felt for a time that Justin needed to be able to expand and be physical in the hours as he was so constrained in the world. Over time, I also began to see the physical play as avoidant of his fears and so not really play. With the final giant crash, I decide a limit is in order for the benefit of Justin, my downstairs neighbor and myself. A play space is also a bounded space. Some boundaries are needed to allow the

possibility of really free play. I will return to this point in the Discussion to speculate where limits within a session may be necessary in other perseverative states in
children or adults in order to try to convey a hope of greater meaning.

### Robots and Fear of Psychosis

In the next part of the hour (Robots and Fear of Psychosis), things do indeed
become more meaningful. The robot material, in part, reflects Justin's wish to be
inanimate and thus not overwhelmed with terror. His robot self also reflects his
experience of having felt inanimate during medical procedures – hooked up to
machines and tubes, unconscious or delusional at times. His play conveyed a sense
that he had had near-death experiences and confusion as to whether he had actually
died or was now someone else. For a tiny child to have to ponder and fear death is
overwhelming. I felt fear during this part of the hour that Justin could be in the grip
of a psychotic process (in Bion's (1967/1957) use of the term) more virulent than
I had thought. Sharing Justin's fears of losing his life is also part of treating him,
inhabiting a fearful or hopeless state and continuing to try to understand. The play
in this part of the hour – of being a robot – seems crucial and close to emotionally
explosive. It is not at all clear Justin is playing at being a robot instead of really
feeling he is a robot. This play space is on the verge of a nightmare.

Aspects of mother's anxiety may have infiltrated Justin in infancy or during
his illnesses (Anzieu-Premmereur, personal communication, 2020). Of course, any
parent would be terribly frightened when their child is having febrile seizures. However, this mother was clear that she had had severe anxiety regarding her mother's
recurrent miscarriages, which likely magnified her fear of Justin's death. Given her
possibly dissociative terror, mother may have been experienced by Justin during
his illness "as a mechanical figure unable to receive and transform his disorganiza-
tion, a non-permeable maternal object, acting like a robot" (Anzieu-Premmereur,
personal communication, 2020, 5). Likewise, my introducing the upcoming break
at the point I was feeling ominous may have reflected a countertransference withdrawal echoing mother's withdrawal when overwhelmed. My ability to fully grasp
mother's likely intense anxiety and drastic defenses during Justin's illness may
have been hampered (ironically) by my experience of her warmth with Justin and
her steady support of his analysis. In other words, I didn't really have a felt experience of overwhelming projected anxiety or inaccessibility in my experience with
this mother that can be quite palpable from some parents.

Given Justin's hatred of noise, it is interesting that the robot needs earpieces to
amplify sound in case someone is trying to kill it. Justin is trapped in a sort of terrible
oversensitivity that is also felt to be necessary because of the dangers around him.
This shows Justin's inhabiting/living a robot state that necessarily breaks down into
fearful paranoia, reminiscent of the mouse that needs to stay away from being sensed
by the snake or lion. Hypersensitivity is felt as necessary and is itself torturous.

After Justin mentions that he would want to hear if someone was trying to kill
him, I interpret: *I was thinking of how you were afraid you were going to die, or*

*maybe it's like you feel a part of you did die – like a part of you is now robot.* As I said earlier, though he did not respond to this interpretation, I felt he understood it and had not just blocked me out as he sometimes does. After this interpretation, he moves to the monsters. I could speculate that my understanding that part of him feels dead or inanimate allowed him to feel somewhat more alive, even if inhabiting a monster world full of dangerous teeth. I next mention that the teeth of the monsters remind me of his having been bitten by his classmate. At the time, I was thinking of how this material might represent his traumatic experience of his classmate's dangerous, attacking teeth coming at him. Retrospectively, I could also wonder if his pre-existing nightmare of being ripped open by the lumbar puncture, etc., was replayed in the biting incident. His phantasy that by being still he can evade danger, may also para-doxically evoke it. The other child may have felt him to be passive and defenseless. Certainly, his phantasy of being invisible does not help him to parry the dangers of the world in the way more active children can. The wish to be invisible can also inter-fere with the sense of a visible self in Winnicott's sense of 'going on being.'

### Teeth and the Ebb and Flow of the Healthy and the Disturbed

In the next part of the hour (Teeth and the Ebb and Flow of the Healthy and the Disturbed), things shift. I felt surprised to notice that despite all the material about teeth, it had never occurred to me whether Justin had lost a tooth. When I asked him, he responded in a way that felt very similar to any healthy child's reaction to these developments. It is exciting and disturbing to lose a part of one-self as one's body grows. He sounded appropriately anxious and proud. He was able to talk to me in a very normal back-and-forth way. I was struck and relieved by the ebb and flow of this so-normal material from my earlier eerie feeling. I was relieved to see the normal so soon after, fearing Justin could be trapped in a terrible psychotic experience. It was interesting to see this relatively fast move-ment from inanimate or horrific material to a far more integrated level of anxiety. That is, he seemed (like most children) to feel anxiety at losing a part of himself, but also with some sense of transitional space – that he could know and not know that other body parts were intact. He also seemed able to feel the progressive part of this bodily change.

### Drawing

Finally, I would like to comment on the intermediate space of drawing with chil-dren in treatment. I found drawing to allow the most potential space of any play modality Justin and I have engaged in. Ferro comments,

> [T]he drawing can be regarded as a sort of "dream-like snapshot of the waking state", which photographs a relational, affective truth . . . . It is a collection of ingredients for possible stories, a source for tales, a "pre-text" requiring reverie and narration.

(1999, 22)

As I have said, Justin seems frightened a great deal of the time. When he tells me about actual nightmares, he is quickly overwhelmed as if the nightmare is really happening. Putting the monsters on paper seems to allow them to be much more under his control than verbalizing them alone. The monsters are literally captured on the page. Whereas at times, Justin's nightmare states left him at the mercy of terrifying psychic reality, in drawing, Justin had the experience of creative aggression – he could make the world. This seems in sync with Winnicott's ideas about the development of a True Self – that is, one has to have self-experiences that are not just compliant or terrified but of creating the world.

One could also see many of Justin's drawings as evacuative – trying to get rid of something overwhelmingly fearful, which is unmetabolized and thus prone to repetition. Indeed, some of Justin's drawings did have a repetitive quality. Yet, Meltzer (1983) suggests the 'fixing' of a fearful drawing on a page is a sort of "fixing of the geography," which may "be the first step in the operation of [in Bion's terms] alpha function" (121).

This 'geographical fixing' with Justin was quite important. He was always startled by noises coming from the street outside my office, which otherwise I might barely notice. I often tried to get him to elaborate on what he thought the sounds might be or imagine aloud myself what the sounds evoked. One day, I merely said, "Justin, the sounds are coming from *outside* the office." He seemed greatly relieved, implying that his sense of inside and outside had been quite confused. His awareness of an inside and outside may at times have been established, but under states of intense fear, he may have collapsed, with no sense of an inside protected by layers of outsides.

Marion Milner, writing in the Winnicottian tradition, discusses how creative play and drawing are integral to change in analysis for her child and adult patients. Halton-Hernandez (2022) describes Milner as seeing the act of making a picture as providing an "attuned, reciprocal relationship with another." Milner coined the term the 'pliable medium' in her 1950 book *On Not Being Able to Paint* (Milner, 2010). She commented that paint "because it does not intrude its demands, but just waits, submitting to things done to it, it does for the painter, I believed, some of the things that a good mother does for her baby" (Milner, 1987, 108).

Molinari (2013), in considering the group nature of the field in child analysis, uses children's drawings to try to establish a method of thinking with parents by sharing their child's drawings that imply implicit situations in the family. Her point is to develop a communicative situation with the parents in the parent work and in the family itself. She emphasizes the importance of the child's drawings both in condensing (as in a dream) elements of the group unconscious – including the analyst as now a member of the field. Molinari suggests that the child's drawings also entail intense contact with bodily experiences, including unconscious ones.

## Conclusion

Winnicott contends that play is immensely exciting, not primarily because the instincts are involved, but because of the "precariousness of the interplay of personal psychic reality and the experience of control of actual objects" (1971, 47).

Justin's fears of being dead, which frequently overwhelmed him, could be represented by him as he drew the half-human/half-robot character. This allowed a new feeling of representability (albeit rigid) to be integrated with existing fears. Drawing allowed him some feeling of control. Being active in creating the drawings allowed him some sense of doing instead of being done to, as well as a sense of safety in terms of locating the monsters on the paper. Still, the nightmare was close enough at hand that I began to have an eerie feeling. The play allowed me to help carry the disturbed feeling for a time, leaving Justin access to his use of play to imagine his own experience.

I would like to return to my limit on Justin's perseverative jumping crashes. I imagine that he could not himself easily decide he was getting bored with something and turn to something else. I could speculate that to notice an absence or a vacancy could feel like an uncharted hole to Justin and that the repetition gave him a feeling of predictability and continuity. A pause may feel like the terrifying 'black hole' Tustin describes, which she sees as an awareness of body separateness that can be experienced as a loss of part of the body, leaving a 'hole' (2021/1992, 82). I may have had to introduce the holes or shifts in some way to help create the experience that they could be survived. While the hole did allow terrors and wishes of being dead in for Justin (and for me in my fear of psychosis), we could also experience together that he did survive.

When treating this boy, I suggested to the parents that he could be at the very high end of Autism Spectrum Disorder (ASD) and recommended a neuropsychological evaluation. (He had evidenced an overwhelmed reaction to sound from earliest times, which could have been contributed to by chaotic experiences during his emergency C-section or may also have represented a neurological vulnerability.) While I think mother might have been open to my recommendation, father was not, and my pushing it further could have alienated father and undermined the alliance that allowed this important work to be done. Just as ASD involves a spectrum of severity, so may some children have some sub-diagnosable element of ASD.

Earlier, I suggested that true play is the precursor of truly free association, and likewise, we could say that perseverative non-play and nightmare states must likewise be precursors of problematic non-free associative states. I will comment here briefly on an adult version of such a non-free associative state. David, an adult male patient, characteristically presented me with a firehose of words, as well as unceasing shifts from topic to topic. Such a flood of words (like Justin's perseverative play) may feel familiar to such a patient and may be felt to block something more catastrophic from happening. But when must we help patients to pause in the face of overwhelming repetition? In such a state, play or a free-association has broken down. In such moments, the analyst must be guided by the sense that our goal is to be able to help a patient return to or attain a play/free-associative state. After an extended period of being barraged by words from David, I told him that I knew there were horrors inside that felt so urgent to get out. And yet, we needed to be able to pause *to think* in order not to be endlessly trapped in the horrors but to have some way to begin to wrap our minds around them. Needless to say, any such process of helping the patient and the patient/analyst pair to move from perseveration or nightmare to playing and free-associating is an ongoing endeavor. The analyst and patient struggling together with the experience of a pause can be part of moving through painful emotions rather than simply analyzing them. Such are the considerations of the establishment of a play space with both adult and child psychoanalytic work.

## Acknowledgments

An earlier version of this chapter was presented at the American Psychoanalytic Association Meetings in New York on February 15, 2020.

## Notes

1  Winnicott saw the "illusion of omnipotence'" (1953, 90) as necessary for the infant, which is provided by the mother so that the infant can feel like God. Winnicott saw this experience as fundamental for a nascent self, but also thought that eventually the process of disillusionment would also have to be facilitated by mother. In a similar vein, Milner used the term illusion to convey that there is no meaning in life without the self's inner contribution to perception.
2  Anzieu stresses containment (or what he terms 'wrapping') of emotions and primitive anxiety over the content of the phantasies.

## References

Alvarez, A. (2012). *The Thinking Heart: Three Levels of Psychoanalytic Therapy with Disturbed Children*. London & New York, NY: Routledge.
Anderson, R. (1997). The child in the adult: The contribution of child analysis to the psychoanalysis of adults. In *The contemporary Kleinians of London* (pp. 414–425). Madison, CT: International Universities Press, Inc.
Anzieu, D. (2016). *The Skin Ego*, trans. Naomi Segal. Karnac. (Original work published 1985.)
Anzieu-Premmereur, C. (2020). Discussion of 'The play's the thing: From nightmare world to play space in a five-year-old'. Unpublished paper presented at the *American Psychoanalytic Association Meetings*, February 15, 2020, New York.
Bion, W.R. (1967). Differentiation of the psychotic from the non-psychotic personalities. In *Second Thoughts* (pp. 43–64). New York: Aronson. (Original work published 1957.)
Elise, D. (2018). A Winnicottian field theory: Creativity and the erotic dimension of the analytic field. *Fort da*, 24(1), 22–38.
Ferro, A. (1999). *The Bi-Personal Field: Experiences in Child Analysis*. London & New York, NY: Routledge.
Halton-Hernandez, E. (2022). Marion Milner's 'pliable medium' and the role of the patient's creativity in the analytic encounter. *British Journal of Psychotherapy*, 38, 433–443.
Mayes, L., & Cohen, D. (1993). Playing and therapeutic action in psychoanalysis. *International Journal of Psychoanalysis*, 74, 1235–1244.
Meltzer, D. (1983). *Dream-Life: A Re-Examination of the Psycho-Analytical Theory and Technique*. Perthshire: Clunie Press.
Milner, M. (1987). *The Suppressed Madness of Sane Men: Forty-Four Years of Exploring Psychoanalysis*. London: Routledge.
Milner, M. (2010). *On Not Being Able to Paint*. London: Routledge. (Original work published 1950.)

Molinari, E. (2013). The use of drawings to explore dual group analytic field in child analysis. *The International Journal of Psychoanalysis*, 94, 293–312.

Parsons, M. (2000). *The Dove that Returns, the Dove that Vanishes*. New York: Taylor and Francis, Inc.

Tustin, F. (2021). *Autistic States in Children*. London & New York, NY: Routledge. (Original work published 1992.)

Winnicott, D.W. (1953). Transitional objects and transitional phenomena: A study of the first not-me possession. *The International Journal of Psychoanalysis*, 34, 89–97.

Winnicott, D.W. (1971). *Playing and Reality*. London: Tavistock Publications.

Chapter 8

# Totalitarian Regimes and a Child's Mind

## Cría Cuervos

*Mary T. Brady, Adriana Prengler, Ana Belchior Melícias and Virginia Ungar*

Spanish director Carlos Saura's[1] (1976) masterpiece *Cría Cuervos* is used here to describe the way violence and repression, enforced by a totalitarian regime, affect the mind – not only for those of the immediate generation but also the next. Faimberg (2005) writes that transmission between generations (both political and personal) is an 'invisible' object in psychoanalyses that needs to be constructed or made visible in film. We will argue here that through art, Saura makes the enforced silence as well as the violence of totalitarian regimes visible as it is transmitted into the film's characters and partially transformed in Ana, the central character of this film.

Eight-year-old Ana (played by then 10-year-old Ana Torrent) believes she killed her dead father (played by Héctor Alterio) and is frequently visited by hallucinations of her dead mother (portrayed by Geraldine Chaplin). Saura vividly depicts the way children's fragile psyches are frozen in time by trauma, here particularly the personal history of the excruciating illness and death of Ana's mother. *Cría* thus also explores the interpenetration of the past and the present when time has been fractured by a traumatic loss.

The interpenetration of reality and fantasy is brilliantly played out in the opening sequence of *Cría Cuervos*. In a white nightgown, Ana descends a dark staircase. As the camera focuses on her pale, expressionless face, urgently whispered adult words – "I love you;" "I can't breathe" – are heard from behind a closed door. A half-dressed woman runs from the room. On entering the now silent room, Ana finds her father in bed, apparently dead. Impassive, she takes a glass to the kitchen and washes it in the sink. As she opens the refrigerator, her mother comes into the shot and addresses her tenderly. Only later do we learn her mother had died some time ago.

The psychological and the political are inextricable in *Cría Cuervos*. The title refers to a Spanish proverb: *"Cría Cuervo y te sacarán los ojos"* ("Raise ravens and they will tear your eyes out"). Ana's father was a Fascist military officer, so the film's title implies a legacy of political and personal violence. Thus, Saura foregrounds in the choice of title the violence that is generated by one generation that will be vengefully returned by the following generation. Saura conveys what Bollas (1992) has discussed psychoanalytically – that fascism is a pathological state of mind as well as a political phenomenon.

DOI: 10.4324/9781003498810-9

Saura shot *Cría Cuervos* in the summer of 1975 as Spanish dictator Francisco Franco lay dying. The film premiered in Madrid in 1976, 40 years after the beginning of the Spanish Civil War, and received the Special Jury Prize at the 1976 Cannes Film Festival.

Saura's early films were heavily censored by the Franco regime and contributed to his development of a metaphorical style. Ironically, the censors' insistence on cutting Saura's films "of specific social, political and historical references left his characters in a vacuum that, with powerful irony, was wholly representative of Saura's view of contemporary Spain as a place of fear, denial and falsehood" (Stone, 2002, 69).

Ana seems a wise child (Ferenczi, 1955) who has witnessed personal, familial, and cultural disasters, grasping the violence and beauty of life (albeit infused by a child's magical and omnipotent thinking). Ana could be seen, in part, as motivated by the epistemophilic instinct, or in other words, the desire to understand. In Bion's view, the desire to understand fundamental emotional truths is more central than the pleasure principle.[2] For instance, Ana is willing to face her Aunt Paulina's disapproval when she refuses to kiss her father in his coffin – reflecting her insistence on emotional truth.

Ana is also motivated by revenge: she has tried to kill her father, whom she holds responsible for the death of her mother due to his cruelty and infidelity. Ana did not actually cause his death, nor is her father literally responsible for her mother's cancer, yet in Ana's child's mind, both are true. Her actions exceed typical childish murderous wishes. Ana mixes a powder that she thinks is poisonous into father's drink and then clearly thinks she has been successful in killing him. She later kindly offers this powder to her grandmother whom she thinks wants to die. She later tries to murder Aunt Paulina with the powder and, this time, is surprised to find that she is unsuccessful. Thus, Ana has imbibed the murderousness of her father and his Francoist regime, although unlike him, she is multi-dimensional and capable of great sensitivity as well. In this sense, she is not overall in a fascist state of mind with a central preoccupation with violence and power, but an element of her father's murderousness is present.

Sabbadini's (2014) commentary on this film emphasizes Ana's preoccupation with death.[3] Child analysts are aware of the way children are often occupied with the great mysteries of life, including death, in ways many adults do not take seriously. Ana's preoccupation with mortality has been intensified by witnessing the deterioration and death of her mother, as well as by her own murderous wishes.

*Cría*'s Ana is a child of great intuition who takes in her personal and cultural surroundings at a depth and judges it unsparingly. Saura said:

*Cría Cuervos* is a sad film, yes. But that's part of my belief that childhood is one of the most terrible parts in the life of a human being. What I'm trying to say is that at that age you've no idea where it is you are going, only that people are taking you somewhere, leading you, pulling you and you are frightened. You don't know where you're going or who you are or what you are going to do.

(quoted by Stone, 2001, 102)

Children *are* absorbed with understanding some of the darkest mysteries of life and are dependent on those around them to protect them from terrible experiences of helplessness, but Saura's childhood was also darkened by growing up in Madrid during the Spanish Civil War. Stone (98) cites Saura's biographer, Enrique Brasó, who quotes Saura:

> I suppose that for Proust his childhood was a series of details more or less poetic of his family and surroundings; for me those memories are much more violent: it's a bomb that falls on my school and a little girl bloodied with shards of glass in her face. And that's no literary invention, it's a fact.
>
> (Brasó, 1974, 23)

Saura was born in 1932 in the Republican-controlled capital of Madrid, which was under siege by Franco from 1936–1939. During the Spanish Civil War, Madrid became a symbol of anti-fascist resistance, enduring a two-and-a-half-year siege, fighting against the rebel forces led by Franco. Madrid was the first major city in history to experience aerial bombardments of its residential neighborhoods and civilians, which was ordered by Franco as punishment. The bombardment was aided by German and Italian aircraft to extinguish the Republican resistance (Bordes & De Sobrón, 2021). Madrid fell to Nationalist forces on March 28, 1939. On April 1, the Republican Army surrendered in all of Spain. After the fall of Madrid, Franco conducted mass punishment and purging of the defeated, and poverty was a punishment "handed out to the vanquished zone" (Stone, 2002, 61).

The great Spanish directors of this period, Luis Buñuel, Victor Erice, and Saura, have created narratives that allow us to reflect and represent the silence and violence of the Franco era. Buñuel denounced fascist power that felt totally justified and approved, destroying freedom. He likewise aimed his criticism at the Catholic Church in Spain, for instance, in his 1961 *Viridiana*. Buñuel managed to largely evade the Spanish censors in this satirical and absurdist film, which, when shown, provoked outrage from the Catholic Church and was then banned in Spain until after Franco's death.

Erice's masterpiece *The Spirit of the Beehive* (1973), set in Spain in 1940, chronicles Spain's isolation and silence under fascism, as well as the marginalization of intellectuals. Like Saura's *Cria*, this film also evaded the Spanish censors by using a metaphorical style but vividly conveyed the silence and violence of its fascist period.[4]

Just as psyches are frozen in time by trauma, one might see *Cría* as Saura's commentary on the potential for a social structure to be traumatized and frozen. Analysts of children, adolescents, and adults must struggle to think in analytic fields dominated by non-thinking states engendered by trauma and splintered by dissociation and splitting. Trauma (including societally, economically, and culturally induced trauma) overwhelms the psyche, while both psychoanalysis and artistic creations such as film allow the psyche to make meaning of trauma. Children and adolescents are often the group most affected by cultural changes and catastrophes.

They are like the canaries sent into coal mines to signal the presence of gases, imbibing cultural, societal, and economic changes in a rapid and powerful way.

We will use the axes of characters, spaces, and settings, as well as memory, to think psychoanalytically of the effects of personal trauma, as well as a totalitarian regime's political violence and enforcement of repressive silence, on the current and succeeding generations.

## The Axis of Characters

In addition to 8-year-old Ana, the other characters in the film are her mother, Maria, her father, Anselmo, her 11-year-old sister, Irene, her 5-year-old sister, Maite, and their grandmother. Rosa, the maid, and Paulina, the aunt (who comes to take care of the girls after both their parents die) complete the household. The final characters are a couple – Amelia (with whom the father is making love when he dies) and her officer husband Nicolas (who becomes the lover of Aunt Paulina).

The viewer is immersed in the darkness of Ana's family, a metaphor for the external socio-political situation. Entrenched authoritarianism is not only relevant to government; it can shape society, mold the family, and impose itself on the structure of the mind.

Anselmo, the military father, can be thought of as representing the Franco regime. He is the powerful dictator in his home, symbolic of oppression, abuse, and intolerance of the other. He follows his own desires without considering any-one else's wishes. He submits others to his will. As a dictator, he needs to remain in power, command others without limits, exclude the other, devalue them, and sub-jugate them into dependence. Anselmo mirrors Franco at the socio-political level. The others in the family cannot escape and have no choice but to submit to their father's authoritarian will.

Maria, the mother, suffers from a terminal illness. She is weak, powerless, and trapped. She can be seen as representing the sick, mistreated, and dying Spain and its oppressed, humiliated people. She is 'Mother Land,' without the attention or love she needs until she dies. Submitted and powerless before her husband, she begs for care and love, as the submitted Spanish society does under the Franco regime. Authoritarianism not only submits the people to dictatorial rule but also justifies their persecution by blaming them. Similarly, Anselmo blames his wife for being annoying and not letting him live happily (in his view, without any restric-tions or responsibilities), thus justifying his actions. This is consonant with Bol-las's assertion that: "the Fascist mind transforms a human other into a disposable non-entity" (1992, 203).

As mentioned previously, Ana blames her father for the suffering of her mother, and this awakens her patricidal desire. Her patricidal impulse, rather than an intra-psychic oedipal conflict, seems to be an effort to avenge the mistreatment her mother received from her husband, Anselmo. It is also an assertion of Ana's own desire for freedom. Ana decides to kill her father with a substance she thinks is poisonous but is really baking soda. Ana can be seen as a raven in relation to the titular proverb. Her attempt to murder her father can also be seen as an effort to be rid of him in order to free herself. We can see her attempted murder of her father as symbolic of the desire of the humiliated Spanish people to eliminate the tyrant who oppresses them, often with an ineffective weapon.

Ana silently witnesses her father's infidelity and his subsequent death. As his lover Amelia runs from the bedroom, Ana's gaze meets Amelia's eyes, and they stare at each other, not as woman and girl but as if they were two women cognizant of the truth about a man. At this moment, Ana loses her childish innocence forever. Surely, this scene confirms something that Ana already knew about Amelia. But from that moment on, Ana and Amelia share a secret. Eventually, Ana (through her sister Irene) dares to reveal to her Aunt Paulina that her father was with Amelia when he died, possibly in an attempt to break the unspoken alliance with Amelia. This can also be seen as the way truth is not accepted in a repressive regime, but it may eventually come to light.

Paulina silences her, forcing her to deny what she has seen with her own eyes: "You did not see anything." Paulina silences the truth and forces Ana to go against her own perception. This can be seen as a mandate to submit to authority without thinking, without speaking, forcing Ana into a disavowal of the truth.

Ana's internal world suffered the same vicissitudes as the external world under Franco's dictatorship. If you tell the truth, you will be punished or killed. In a totalitarian regime, there is no place for the truth, for freedom of expression, for sharing, for healthy alliances.

The three generations, Ana, her mother, and her grandmother, are forced into the fate that has befallen them. They are not to speak. This is epitomized by the grandmother, who literally *does not speak*. She only dreams while listening to the music of her past and looking at the photos that remind her of a happier time long, long ago. The three generations suffer fear, uncertainty, threat, confusion, loneliness, helplessness, and hopelessness at home and societally. Once again, Ana must submit to silence and an imposition, now from her aunt. Ana's wish to kill her aunt may reflect her rage at her aunt for replacing her mother, but also her belief that it is better to kill her aunt and attain some freedom. Both father and aunt, in different ways, represent the abuse of power and the disconnection of affection.

In one compelling flashback, Ana sees her mother screaming in pain on her deathbed. This scene conveys Ana's impotence and sadness. It is analogous to the impotence and the pain in Spanish society, which was traumatized and frozen in fear, as is Ana's gaze in this scene. Ana is wordless as she sees her mother die. She looks off into space, paralyzed, and expressionless. She does not feel entitled to hug her mother or talk to her on her deathbed. How will she be able to mourn this terrible loss? The scene can be thought of as conveying how difficult it is to grieve for someone one hasn't been able to say goodbye to, as in the cases of those who have been disappeared by a repressive regime. As in a frightening dictatorship, there is no one to talk to and no one to trust.

Ana feels guilty for having 'killed' her father and for wanting to kill her aunt with her poisonous baking soda. The poison conveys the rage that Ana feels and yet has no right to express openly. In one scene, Ana tells her doll, "You're bad!" projecting onto the doll her guilt for having in fantasy murdered her father and having tried to kill her aunt. In a subsequent scene, Ana plays a version of hide and seek with her sisters, in which those found must fall to the ground 'dead.' They play at dying and being resurrected, perhaps with the wish to resurrect their mother. One can see the attempt to make representable what is unrepresentable about death. One can also see the link that Ana makes between killing and dying, which is so characteristic of childhood games. At the time of filming in 1975, Spain's freedom had long been dying, but there was hope that it would soon be resurrected.

At one point in the film, Ana asks her grandmother, "Do you want me to help you die?" Ana, also, in part, seems to have wished to die. There is a repetitive, bizarre image in the film of a plate of chicken feet seen when Ana opens the refrigerator. When made into soup, chicken feet are a common home remedy for many ailments. Chicken feet can also be an amulet for protection and good luck, counteracting bad energy. They stay fresh in the refrigerator, ready to be used as if they are the source of magical hope. The film seems to leave in question how much Ana can meaningfully, psychically recover, and survive (e.g., with the help of the chicken feet) or whether this is just a magical idea in the face of overwhelmingly harsh realities.

Ana is a victim of a terrible family situation in which she is submerged. She knows that she should hide herself, hide the poison, hide the truth – not only the material poison but the poison of pain and anger. She watches and 'kills' without any expression. Ana hides her 'crimes,' as dictatorial regimes do, trying to keep up appearances, just like her father Anselmo, who goes to church and then unsuccessfully hides his relation to his lover.

Near the end of the film, Irene, the older sister, tells Ana her nightmare, in which kidnappers threatened to kill her. Irene finishes her story with the following words: "[T]hey put a gun to my temple, and when they were going to kill me . . . I woke up." In her dream, she was tied up, abused, not able to talk, submissive and scared. Of the three sisters, Irene is the one who tries to adapt to the tyrant, to be obedient, to try not to get in trouble. Her dream seems to express her underlying experience of defenselessness, her uncertainty about her survival, and her hope that she won't be killed.

Psychoanalysis looks for the 'truth' of the patient, with all the consequences that it may bring. What is unconscious is made conscious. In a dictatorial system, the opposite occurs. The regime tries to deny truth and disavow reality. Being raised in a dictatorial system shapes the mind. The possibility of being severely punished, rejected, or killed makes it difficult to differ from publicly mandated 'truths.' It takes years or perhaps generations to trust that thinking differently from leadership will not be punished by death or exclusion.

Ana suffers experiences that will take decades to repair – if she succeeds at all. There is a similar challenge for a society casting off the cloak of oppression. A denied trauma is never forgotten because it remains ready to be repeated. As Freud would say, we need to remember trauma to be able to forget it and avoid repeating it. It seems that the compulsion to repeat occurs not only individually but also at the level of societies in wars, dictatorships, killings, and discrimination. Internal and external realities are imbricated.

## The Axis of Spaces and the Axis of Memory

In this section, we will discuss another element of the film – that of spaces and settings. External spaces are intimately interconnected with internal spaces in *Cría*, similar to how collective history contains the individual. Another axis of the film is memory, as a potential space for transformation. Saura, in resistance to dictatorship, makes full use of fantasy. He creates films between the psychological and the political, between the feminine and the masculine, childhood, adulthood, and old age, vulnerability and violence, and freedom and oppression. Ana personifies remaining connected to psychic reality – both to her process of mourning and loss, as well as to the positive and loving relations that she insists on remembering. She rejects narratives imposed on her that she knows are not true. Daydreaming and playing allow her to resist, actively acting out what she suffers passively (*fort-da*).

The mansion (in which most of the film is set) is enclosed by high walls, like a bunker, a non-home. It could be thought of as representing a totalitarian space of mind – a space of confinement and dictatorship, a space of negative links and psychotic parts of the mind (Bion, 1962/1984), such as hypocrisy, betrayal, violence, and arrogance. The mansion is in contrast to Bachelard's concept of the house: "[T] he house shelters daydreaming, the house protects the dreamer, the house allows one to dream in peace" ([1969] 1989, 26). The interior spaces of the mansion are suffused with darkness and shadow, reflecting anguish and pain. Ana dreams of a liberating flight from the silent and gloomy mansion-dictatorship to the vitalized, almost deafening noise of Madrid. In one scene, she stands on the roof of the mansion, but she does not fall; she imagines herself flying, as often happens in children's dreams.

The paralysis and dependency represented by grandmother's wheelchair convey involuntary imprisonment: lack of freedom of movement and speech, as well as silencing of communication and dialogue. Conversely, Ana has the most intimate and empathetic relationship with her paralyzed grandmother, who is dependent and unable to speak. Ana remains internally connected to loving links – her guinea pig, her sisters, her grandmother, and Rosa the maid – remembering the warm embrace of her mother(land) through piano music and bedtime stories.

Ana's true and deep gaze entails a:

(D)ouble movement of looking outward and seeing inward. A wise child, Ana speaks little but observes and listens a lot, vigilant to external noises as well as internal ones, in search of knowledge.

(Melícias, 2021)

Ana lovingly cares for her guinea pig, Roni, who is in a cage space with a wheel. Her lovingly feeding Roni lettuce can be seen in contrast to being in a cage on a repetitive autocratic wheel-mind preventing creativity and relationships.

The parents' room/bed, instead of representing a primal loving scene space, is linked to the painful memory of the mother's agonizing illness. The room/bed is also linked to witnessing the father's betrayal and to the father's death – desired and magically achieved in fantasy.

On the other hand, the children's room presents itself as a vitalized and potential space (Winnicott, 1971/1975) for experience. In one scene, the three children playfully act out the arguments they have heard between the parents. In one scene, the children imitate interchanges overheard from their parents. Their healthy sororal complicity allows their staging of the (non)love of their parents. Femininity also blossoms as they investigate and play with women's magazines, makeup, dances, and love songs, preparing for adolescence. The sororal dimension is decisive in many traumatic situations as well as in resistance groups and organized struggle. But the children's room also houses fears of the night, darkness, nightmares, and mourning so painful to process. Winnicott warns us that: "[T]here is a limited value to internal freedom . . . if it is consciously experienced only in persecutory circumstances" (1969/1989, 185).

The setting of the unsettlingly empty swimming pool in the backyard implies the absence of the uterine aquatic womb and instead can be seen as tomblike. This space without content becomes occupied by Ana, in which she builds a hut. She keeps alive the capacity for 'make believe' that is necessary for the elaboration of reality, from passively experienced to actively imagined. Through playing with the dolls/infants, Ana elaborates on internal conflicts, processing ambivalence toward a good and bad mother. But, the authoritarian aggressor can be seen here as well in her superegoic games of punishment and guilt, negating vulnerability and difference. Ana's play and creativity fill the empty pool, transforming the claustrophobic emptiness and dehumanization of authoritarian regimes.

Contrasting with this negative space where she conveys her 'capacity to be alone' (Winnicott, 1958), Ana feels accompanied by Rosa in the kitchen, an ancestral-oral space of nourishment. The kitchen is a primary space of concreteness but also a space of curiosity about the mysteries of origin and birth. With Rosa, she learns prosaically and without taboos about men, love, betrayal, disease, death, and birth. With Rosa, she quenches her curiosity about her own birth. She also asks to see Rosa's breasts and satisfies her voyeurism, surprising herself when she sees Rosa's big breast – both erotic and nourishing.

We now turn to the bathroom – a space of secrets and taboos. It is in the bathroom that Ana reveals her secret to Aunt Paulina that her father died while having sex with Amelia. Aunt Paulina then insists it isn't true, teaching denial and hypocrisy. The bathroom setting is the space of anality *par excellence*, of control and authoritarian power exercised by Aunt Paulina trying to force Ana into a lie.

Perhaps the wall of photos that grandmother and Ana view together iconically represents the entire film. Viewing the photo wall together, Ana empathetically offers to help her grandmother – either to die if she so desires or to live by traveling through her good memories. Sharing memories allows us to surpass the limits of space and time. Memory is also a place to 'go outside inside.' *Cría* begins with Ana's memory album – "the day I was born" – and is a narrative dialogue between Ana as a child and the memories of adult Ana shown in flash-forward scenes. Memory, a generator of thought, is a potential space for freedom, creativity, reparation, and hope.

Memory entails a kind of language of emotion that fosters mourning (breast, mother, father, childhood, countries, relationships, etc.) from which new narratives can be dynamically articulated. New narratives can arise from the use of negative capability (Bion, 1977/2019), including the toleration of doubt, uncertainty, and mystery. Memory can also be a space that can resist manipulative and misleading discourse utilized by totalitarian regimes. Memory, by allowing us to create a new experience, transforms the tragedy of catastrophe into benign catastrophic changes (Bion, 1966) and transforms the fatality of fate into a creative opportunity.

As mentioned earlier, just before the final scene of the film, Irene tells Ana a nightmare as they eat breakfast, "They put a gun to my head, and when they were going to kill me . . . I woke up." Spain and the children wake up from a long nightmare of fascism. In the final scene of the film, the girls emerge from the mansion on their own for their first day back at school. This scene embodies relief and hope. It becomes possible to go outside, away from Francoism and the claustrum-mansion. In the wide space of the freedom of the city street, we follow Irene, Ana, and Maite. They are released from the walls on their way to school, an exogamous space of expansion, knowledge, culture, and enriching affective exchanges.

## Conclusion

Manmade humanitarian catastrophes such as the Holocaust, wars, and political and ethnic persecutions use dehumanization and destruction of subjectivity to annihilate the historical and social existence of individuals and groups. Psychoanalytic work attempts to integrate these traumatic experiences into a narrative context. Collective traumas also require a social discourse on the historical truth of the traumatic events, as well as on their defensive denial.

Psychoanalysis works in the search for truth. If there is censorship in a country, if there is no freedom of expression, if the law does not prevail, and if justice becomes a non-functioning structure, the most profound and essential part of a child's development is threatened. The traumatic effects of lack of freedom appear in the impairment of subjectivity that can be observed analytically. *Cría*'s characters convey the dynamic processes of subjectivization, which occur in the children's interaction with their time.

We live in a world with the ghosts of the past. Today's wars, as well as violence in its various forms, racism, xenophobia, and fanatical leaders, are eloquent proof that the tendency towards human self-destruction is still alive. Films play a key role in creating a reflective space for societal traumas, especially when so much of our lives are spent in virtual reality, and cinema has managed to reach the masses through online platforms. Films can function by intervening, modifying, and interacting with the society that produces them, that is, as agents of history. They set in motion the memories and direct experiences we have of different events. History is superimposed by the images of films, which in this way give additional content to our own images of the past.

The psychoanalytic approach to art and aesthetics has a long tradition. Some approaches focus on the analysis of literary works as a key to biographical studies of their authors. Some study the work of art itself. In relation to the former, *Cria* is a journey through Saura's childhood. The film was released in 1976, at the time that Franco was slowly dying, inaugurating what was called the Transition period in Spain. This historical interval is reflected in the transformation processes of *Cria's* protagonist, Ana. Saura masterfully used a narrative technique that was disoriented with flashbacks and flash-forwards. Present and past situations are shown in a dreamlike manner, leaving unclear what is memory, hallucination, or part of the current narrative. There is a flow of superimposed memories and images, similar to how thoughts and emotions crowd our minds.

Saura created a narrative of great beauty, even within societal and familial horror, in which he manages to blur the boundaries that separate life from death and childhood from adulthood. He did it with a delicate vision, attentive to detail, always seen through Ana's hypnotic gaze.

The creative union of cinema and psychoanalytic thinking is an important agent in the process of construction and support of collective memory. We have hoped to convey here how societal and familial violence, lack of freedom, fear, sadness, and hopelessness deeply affect development and shape a child's vision of the world. *Cria* conveys a sense that Ana will wrestle with these issues for a lifetime, as Saura acknowledges he did himself.

Ana and the sisters (representing childhood) inhabit virtually every scene in the film. They share a similar view of the events that build their lives and yet have unique ways of relating to these events. The spectator is one more child in this same confusing and depressing reality. However, the sisters also share the creativity of play – they kill and resurrect, disguise themselves, dance, and imagine – thus allowing a potential space necessary for life itself.

### Acknowledgments

This chapter was first presented at a panel entitled 'Adolescence in the Line of Fire: Reflections on the Impact of Pandemic and War' at the International Psychoanalytic Association Congress on 'Minds in the Line of Fire,' Cartagena, July 27, 2023.

### Notes

1  Saura also wrote and produced *Cría.*
2  Ambrosio Garcia discusses cinema in Bion's terms as a "thinking space . . . which drives the subject in the search for truth even if it is painful" (2017, 50).

3 Sabbadini also asserts that Saura, (which he sees as rare for male directors), has a deep understanding of female internal worlds. Sabbadini comments that all the central characters in *Cría* are female, and the male characters only marginal.

4 For a current paper on *Beehive*, see Gerhardt and Slobin (2024).

## References

Ambrosio Garcia, C 2017. *Bion in Film Theory and Analysis: The Retreat in Film.* London and New York: Routledge.

Bachelard, G 1969. *The Poetics of Space*, trans. Maria Jolas. Boston: Beacon Press. [(1989). A poética do espaço. São Paulo: Martins Fontes.]

Bion, WR 1962/1984. *Learning from Experience.* London and New York: Karnac.

Bion, WR 1966. Catastrophic change. In: *Bull 5* (Vol. II). British Psychoanalytical Society, pp. 13–26.

Bion, WR 1977/2019. Capacidade negativa. In: *Capacidade Negativa. Um caminho em busca de luz. (Trad. Aile Stürmer).* Zagodoni, pp. 125–135.

Bollas, C 1992. The fascist state of mind. In: *Being a Character: Psychoanalysis and Self Experience.* New York: Routledge.

Bordes, E & De Sobrón, L 2021. *Madrid Bombardeado: Cartografía De La destrucción, 1936 – 1939.* Cátedra.

Brasó, E 1974. *Carlos Saura.* Madrid: Taller de Ediciones Josefina Betantor.

Faimberg, H 2005. *The Telescoping of Generations.* Hove: Routledge.

Ferenczi, S 1955. Confusion of tongues between adults and the child. The language of tenderness and of passion. In: *Final Contributions to the Problems and Methods of Psycho-analysis.* London: Hogarth, pp. 156–167. (Original work published 1933 [1932])

Gerhardt, J & Slobin, D 2024. Victor Erice's film *'The Spirit of the Beehive'*: A coded warning against submission in the aftermath of the Spanish Civil War. *Psan Dialogues*, 34(2).

Melícias, AB 2021. *Blog Cinema & Psicanálise – Totality Is the Non-true – October 2021.* https://cinemapsicanalise.pt/2021/10/06/a-totalidade-e-a-nao-verdade-cria-corvos-1976/.

Sabbadini, A 2014. *Moving Images: Psychoanalytic Reflections on Film.* London and New York: Routledge.

Stone, R 2002. *Spanish Cinema.* Essex, UK: Routledge.

Winnicott, DW 1958/1998. A capacidade para estar só. In: *O ambiente e os processos de maturação.* Porto Alegre: Artes Médicas, pp. 31–37.

Winnicott, DW 1969/1989. A liberdade, In: *Tudo começa em casa.* São Paulo: Martins Fontes, p. 185.

Winnicott, DW 1971/1975. O brincar: uma exposição teórica. In: *O brincar e a realidade.* Rio de Janeiro: Imago, pp. 59–77.

# Chapter 9

# Adolescent Psychic Isolation and Bodily-Based Symptoms in the COVID-19 Pandemic

In this chapter, I consider the effects of the COVID-19 pandemic in the United States on the adolescent developmental process. Beginning in March 2020, the COVID pandemic and response (which included physical distancing, stay-at-home orders and the initiation of on-line school) disrupted daily life in the U.S. Additionally, public health measures to restrict the spread of the virus required psychoanalysts and psychotherapists to shift to on-line teletherapy abruptly.[1] The need for remote treatment resulted in the loss of our usual frames and settings and the need to reimagine how to work with each patient.

Of course, the nature of a pandemic is that the virus does not care about national borders, so infection ran rampant throughout the world. As Ungar says, "This humanitarian tragedy shed light on the failure of the prevailing economic system worldwide. Inequities, inequalities in terms of access to education and health . . . have become more evident" (2024 58).

During the extended COVID pandemic, I found myself little interested in writing or presenting about the psychic effects of the virus or the related restrictions. It was as if I felt COVID was already taking up so much room I could not grant it more of my attention. While confronted with the global, general and public-ness of public policy, I felt more than ever that our efforts to find meaning with our patients is what matters. And yet, as Jacob (a late teen whom I will discuss further on) said after the pandemic precautions loosened, "It feels impossible to really take in how big this was, how much it affected everything." As Shulman notes, during the pandemic, even more than usual,

> a reliance on the therapist's own resources is needed, to preserve hope, faith and creativity or alternatively, to rediscover them in new forms in the therapeutic relationship. All this happens despite the fact that the therapist herself is under the same attack as the one her patients are experiencing.
>
> (2020 297)

There are moments post-pandemic that this episode still feels unreal, both to analysts and to patients – we were in the same tumult. We had to deal with some of the same COVID distance-making protections, such as masks and remote

DOI: 10.4324/9781003498810-10

communication, as well as some of the same emotions, such as worry about becoming infected ourselves, worry about infecting others, the strangeness of empty freeways and the horror of one more news image of an isolated death in an Intensive Care Unit.

In normal adolescence, bodily changes and psychological separation from parents (which are part of the developmental process) can lead to what I have termed painful states of psychic isolation (Brady, 2015), when all that is new cannot be easily expressed or even thought. Although one can experience psychic isolation at any age, it is particularly prevalent in adolescence for developmental reasons. I regard psychic isolation in adolescence as an affective state with important developmental underpinnings. The affective experiences are estrangement, loneliness and sometimes a feeling of freakishness. The developmental underpinnings include shifting (conscious as well as unconscious, internal as well as external) object relations and senses of the self. While developmentally normal, psychic isolation can leave the adolescent cut off from others who might be psychically containing, relegating his or her body as the likely receptacle for troubles. I picture Amelia, a 15-year-old I worked with on the phone during COVID. Her bedroom was in the basement of her home – which she liked in general – as it gave her some distance from her parents. But I remember the feeling of strangeness picturing her in the basement, cut off from her regular school and friends and speaking of how dysregulated her eating and sleeping were. If she snuck out for some in-person time with friends, she was left worried about infecting her parents or grandparents. This pandemic added additional levels of strangeness and isolation to Amelia's existing feelings of freakishness at her body and her uncertain sexuality.

As for Amelia, social isolation necessitated by public health measures added to developmental psychic isolation for many teens. Often, this left them to fall back more drastically on their bodies – leading to dysregulated eating and sleeping, as well as hypochondriacal symptoms and the development of some more serious bodily-based syndromes such as eating disorders, substance abuse or suicide attempts.[2]

COVID differentially affected people who are economically disadvantaged and/or ethnic minorities in the U.S. For instance, over 200,000 parents in the U.S. died of COVID during the pandemic. These deaths fell to a much greater degree on low-income People of Color, who often were not able to leave in-person work.[3] As De Rementeria (2020) cogently comments in her introduction to a special section on the pandemic in *The Journal of Child Psychotherapy*: "[W]hile we are all in the same storm, we are not in the same boat" (2020 270). Shillito (2020) similarly notes the disproportionate impact on adolescents in Brent, an underprivileged borough of London where the Brent Centre for Young People is located, including suffering one of the highest death tolls in the U.K.[4] COVID hardships also, of course, interact with and exacerbate numerous familial, intrapsychic and developmental issues that teens experience.

To examine these issues in greater depth, I will discuss my work with an early adolescent girl and a late adolescent male in relation to the extended COVID crisis.

## Pandora

I began to see 'Pandora,' a Caucasian 10-year-old fifth grader, in twice-weekly psychotherapy in January of 2018. Her family situation was chaotic. Mother had been absent for many months due to her suicide attempt and mental illness. It was not clear at the time if or how mother would return to the family. Father was well-intentioned but highly stressed with two daughters, an absent and mentally ill wife and full-time employment as a scientist. Pandora was depressed, withdrawn at school, obsessed with food and overweight. In an early session, she asked me if her mother was going to die. Two years later, the mother returned to contact with the family when father initiated divorce proceedings. I found mother self-involved, grandiose and highly reactive to any exploration of the effect of her illness or absence on her daughter. But I also thought that Pandora improved as she saw her mother was recovering from the most severe period of mental illness and was going to stay involved with her. At 13, Pandora had just begun to emerge into social relations and the beginning experience of a best friend.

As I mentioned earlier, COVID restrictions differentially affected children depending on economic circumstances. Though father made a good income, he was under financial strain as mother returned and sued for alimony and child support. Pandora attended public school, which in the U.S. shut down for long periods of time, while private schools were often more nimble and resumed in-person learning much more quickly. The San Francisco Public School system shut down from March 16, 2020, through August 2021. Thus, Pandora's last three months of 7th grade were abruptly on-line as well as her entire 8th grade – she never returned to the Middle School she had attended.

Pandora had difficulty concentrating in on-line school, which affected her academic development. Her father was working from home while his two children attended school virtually. I could tell from my collateral on-line sessions with father that his attention was pulled away to work issues coming in on his screen as we talked. I knew that Pandora was suffering from his severely taxed attention. Pandora, likewise, was often late for her on-line sessions, which I interpreted as letting me feel what it was like to be with someone who was half there. She would stick her rear end in the screen or insist that she had to bake during a session, though I knew this would make her minimally available for our work.

Often, she would put on make-up during our sessions, which might sound playful or interactive, but I think was primarily a hostile projective identification – e.g., 'everyone is distracted and unavailable and I will make you feel what that is like.' I interpreted that all of our disappearances from her (losing *our* in-person sessions, as well as her teachers and her friends) made her angry and that she conveyed it to me by not wanting to be present for me. I also thought that she was expressing anger in the transference for her mother's earlier unavailability. However, Pandora was highly sensitive to any comment that could be construed as a criticism of her mother.

Pandora is overweight and has asthma, so her risk factors for a severe experience of COVID were high. I would have liked to return to in-person sessions with her sooner than we did, but Pandora would have had to take public transportation to her sessions and her father understandably felt this was too risky for contracting the virus.

The loss of in-person school seriously retarded Pandora's possibilities for emotional and social development with her peers, capacities which were already lagging. Tyminski (2021) has described how COVID interfered with the adolescent tasks of "adventuring, experimenting and gaining new experiences" (p. 546). In early adolescence, the best friend allows an experience of a couple and the trying on of different possibilities through identifications and idealizations of the friend. Me/not me doesn't have to be clearly defined in this transitional space. While psychic isolation is a normal part of adolescence, teens are unable to try on identifications with peers in an increasingly nuanced manner when they are also literally socially isolated.

The best friend can also help to bridge the anxiety of the leaps required of adolescents, such as that from middle school into high school. Now 15, Pandora entered in-person high school after having lost a year and three months of in-person school. She was not able to negotiate social relations well, leaving her feeling desperate and isolated. Her binge eating disorder had also increased while she was left to manage herself alone during the school day. As Meltzer (1973) rightly comments: "the return of severe splitting processes, characteristic of infancy and early childhood, which attends the adolescent flux, requires externalization in group life so that the omnipotence and confusional states . . . may be worked through" (p. 57). Pandora was deprived of this opportunity at a crucial developmental juncture.

## Jacob

'Jacob,' a Caucasian 19-year-old in analysis when COVID struck, was in some ways aided by the reduced activity necessitated by the pandemic. He had been referred to treatment by his parents at 17 because, while academically highly successful, he barely spoke with them. A few years earlier, he had suffered during a move the family made, which also included the loss of a beloved nanny who died soon after. This move and loss exacerbated his underlying fragility and tendency to narcissistic defenses. He was increasingly withdrawn from his family and chronically angry. Jacob is of exceptional intelligence, as are his rather august parents. His parents had multiple professional and civic responsibilities, and he, as an ambitious teen, had multiple activities.

Early in our work, Jacob treated me as if I was on a retainer. He refused to have a regular standing appointment, and I, at first, decided to see if we might be able to engage what lay under his antagonism to commitment. After a few months of this uncommitted situation, I told him that he was not allowing anyone to be important to him and it would not be useful for us to go on working in this limited way. I told him he could return when he could make a commitment to our work. We stopped at that point, and he called me a few months later. When he started a regular schedule with me, he would still withdraw after meaningful contact and miss sessions, but there was beginning to be an ongoing process. He left for a prestigious college in the Fall of 2019, and we continued sessions on the phone. He told me his mother had referred to a worry that he would kill himself at college. Jacob's social anxiety nearly overwhelmed him in college. He experienced either good or bad emotions coming towards him from others almost more than he could manage.

In March of 2020, when COVID and consequent stay-at-home orders were issued, Jacob was in his second semester of his freshman year at college. He returned home, and the combination of being in analysis and increased time with his parents allowed a turning point. By then, we had worked on his feelings of anger and superiority, as well as his tendency to live in his own world. He was still rather alienated from his parents. During this unexpected period at home due to COVID restrictions, Jacob's parents were traveling less and were less busy with their numerous involvements. One night, while his parents were watching television, he went to their room, got in bed with them and, crying, told them that his outside success was in complete contrast to his internal despair. His parents listened to him and hugged him. This breakthrough seemed the beginning of a move away from his chronic antagonism toward his parents and away from an entrenched narcissistic formation. I was impressed that this family was able to make use of the at-home period to come together and work towards some repair.

On the other hand, as for many adolescents, the emotional pressures of being home without structure contributed to bodily-based symptoms, in his case, binge eating. He told me, "I keep spiraling. It's hard to be at home and not doing anything and be healthy." His dysregulated eating, sleeping and substance use during the COVID isolation seemed an exaggeration of typical adolescent tendencies.

His college allowed half of the students to come back on campus for each of the next two semesters (with virtual classes) and to be in a pod with a few friends. He attended the Fall semester in person. His family has a second home where he and some friends lived during the Spring semester. While such resources are quite an advantage, Jacob also experienced the situation as stressful. He felt substantial internal pressure that his friends be happy and felt quite anxious to be an intermediary between them and his family. While progressing, he was still rather ill-equipped to deal with the feelings this experience entailed.

## Conclusion

I have described psychic isolation in adolescence – an affective state caused by developmental demands. I see the social isolation measures required by COVID as exacerbating these normative issues for many teens. For instance, the cessation of in-person school halted Pandora's already retarded social development and worsened her binge eating. Jacob's experience was less usual as the COVID isolation measures provided meaningful time with his parents, which had been in short supply due to the demands of success as well as his anger at his parents. In conjunction with his analysis, this extra time with his parents allowed significant psychological work to happen. However, he too suffered from the upheavals of COVID in intersection with his nascent capacities to tolerate his own and others' emotions. His binge eating was exacerbated by the lack of external structure and social isolation. These all added to the developmentally normal adolescent difficulty articulating emotions and finding containing minds.

Therapists are often left to wonder. Jacob continued analysis after the pandemic, so I could see his developmental trajectory and his increasing capacity to weather his internal and external worlds. However, Pandora and I stopped working together after the pandemic subsided. Although she returned to meeting with me in the office, she was often late or missed appointments. Coming to my office on her own on buses was harder for her now than when her nanny had brought her when she was younger. But I also wonder about the deleterious effects to our relationship by the limitations of being on-line. As Shillito observes:

> Before Covid-19, remote therapy was something I was aware 'other therapists' practiced. I think it was thought of, not just by me, as a poor relation, a last resort, a temporary contingency. One was exhorted to consider carefully whether a particular patient might be suitable for this way of working and whether it might be better not to work at all with them until such time as they could attend in person. The pandemic changed this: we did not have a choice but to work remotely if sessions were to continue.
>
> (2020 331)

Likewise, pre-pandemic, I would often resist requests for phone sessions, thinking that unconsciously, a patient could experience such a variation as not really holding them close. With COVID, we had little choice, but perhaps the two vignettes presented convey a sense of the varying outcomes for adolescents affected by these COVID disruptions.

## Acknowledgments

This chapter was first presented at a panel entitled 'Adolescence in the Line of Fire: Reflections on the Impact of Pandemic and War' at the International Psychoanalytic Association Congress on 'Minds in the Line of Fire,' Cartagena, July 27, 2023.

## Notes

1 Some papers take up teens' experience of remote therapy, e.g., Benzel and Graneist (2023), Kleinman, Johnston, Dekel and Corn (2023) and MacKean, Lecchi, Mortimer and Midgley (2023), while this chapter discusses the impact of the pandemic and its various resultant changes on the adolescent developmental process.
2 For instance, in the U.S., the C.D.C. (Center for Disease Control) reported (Yard et al., 2021) that the mean weekly number of Emergency Room visits for suspected suicide attempts among those aged 12–17 were 22.3% higher during the summer of 2020 and 39.1% higher during Winter 2021 than during the corresponding periods in 2019, with a more pronounced increase amongst girls. www.who.int/news-room/fact-sheets/detail/suicide

3 For instance, more than twice as many Black children lost a parent than White or Asian children in the U.S., while nearly four times as many American Indian or Alaskan Native children lost a parent than White or Asian children. Hispanic children were 1.5 times more likely to lose a parent than White or Asian children. https://imperialcollegelondon. github.io/orphanhood_USA/

4 See also Rice (2023) in relation to children's experience of parental death during the COVID epidemic.

## References

Benzel, S. & Graneist, A. (2023). "Bye, Click, and Gone" A qualitative study about the experiences of psychotherapists and adolescent patients on remote treatment during the COVID-19 pandemic. *Psychoanalytic Psychology, 40*, 190–198.

Brady, M. T. (2015). 'Unjoined persons': Psychic isolation in adolescence and its relation to bodily symptoms. *Journal of Child Psychotherapy, 41*(2), 179–194.

De Rementeria, A. (2020). Editorial. Journal of Child Psychotherapy, *46*(3), 269–272. https://imperialcollegelondon.github.io/orphanhood_USA/ www.who.int/news-room/fact-sheets/detail/suicide

Kleinman, K., Johnston, M.H., Dekel, N. & Corn, A. (2023). The real, the virtual, and the pandemic. Psychoanalytic Psychology, 40, 199–206.

MacKean, M., Lecchi, T., Mortimer, R. & Midgley, N. (2023). 'I've started my journey to coping better': Exploring adolescents' journeys through an Internet-Based Psychodynamic Therapy (I-PDT) for depression. Journal of Child Psychotherapy, 49, 432–453.

Meltzer, D. (1973). Identification and socialization in adolescence. In *Sexual States of Mind*, pp. 51–57. London: Karnac Books Ltd.

Rice, T. (2023). Children Who Lose a Parent in the COVID-19 Era: Considerations on Grief and Mourning. *The Psychoanalytic Study of the Child, 76*(1), 35–50. https://doi.org/10.1 080/00797308.2022.2120336

Shillito, K. (2020). Reflections on working with adolescents during the Covid-19 pandemic. *Journal of Child Psychotherapy, 46*, 329–335.

Shulman, Y. (2020). The (almost) impossible profession: Face-to-face child psychotherapy during the Covid-19 outbreak. *Journal of Child Psychotherapy, 46*(3), 296–304.

Tyminski, R. (2021). Adolescents coping with the COVID-19 pandemic: 'Every day is like another Sunday'. *Journal of Analytical Psychology, 66*, 546–560.

Ungar, V. (2024). The turbulence of puberty in an uncertain world. In *The Astonishing Adolescent Upheaval in Psychoanalysis*, pp. 54–63. Editors R. Cassorla and S. Flechner. Oxon: Routledge.

Yard, E., Radhakrishnan, L., Ballesteros, M. F., et al. (2021). Emergency department visits for suspected suicide attempts among persons aged 12–25 years before and during the COVID-19 pandemic – United States, January 2019–May 2021. *MMWR Morbidity and Mortality Weekly Report, 70*, 888–894. http://dx.doi.org/10.15585/mmwr.mm7024e1

# Index